Dear family, friends, c[...]
chronic pain sufferers, and Athletes
hampered by injury,

Remember that no matter what happens
in life; no matter how bad the
pain gets — you can always

Prolo Your Pain Away!

Sincerely,

Ross & Marion

Prolotherapy:
An Alternative to Knee Surgery

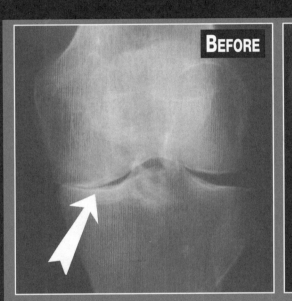 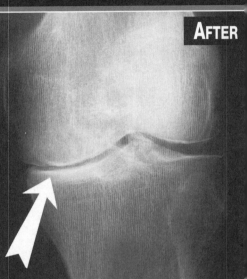

BEFORE · AFTER

Cartilage is regenerated, eliminating "bone-on-bone."

Don't remove your knee tissue— *Re-build it!*

Ross A. Hauser, M.D.
Physical Medicine and Rehabilitation Specialist

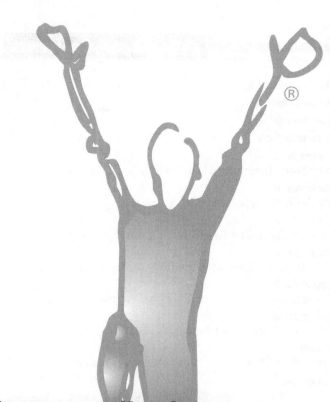

PROLOTHERAPY: AN ALTERNATIVE TO KNEE SURGERY

ISBN 0-9661010-8-1

Text and Illustrations Copyright © 2004, Beulah Land Press
Cover and Page Design Copyright © 2004
Illustrations and Charts by Thomas Penna, M. Hurley, and Joe Faraci

Published by Beulah Land Press
715 Lake Street, Suite 600, Oak Park, Illinois 60301

Printed in the United States of America

Design by Teknigrammaton Graphics
773-973-1614 • Teknigram@ATTGlobal.net
4312 N. Hamilton • Chicago, Illinois 60645

Scripture quotations are from: Holy Bible, New International Version®, NIV®
Copyrights © 1973, 1978, 1984, International Bible Society. Used by permission of Zondervan Publishing House. All rights reserved.

III

TABLE OF CONTENTS

DISCLAIMER

The information presented in this book is based on the experiences of the authors, publishers, and editors, and is intended for informational and educational purposes only. In no way should this book be used as a substitute for your own physician's advice.

Because medicine is an ever-changing science, readers are encouraged to confirm the information contained herein with other sources. The authors, publishers, and editors of this work have used sources they believe to be reliable to substantiate the information provided. However, in view of the possibility of human error or changes in medical sciences, neither the authors, publishers, or editors, nor any other party who has been involved in the preparation or publication of this work warrants that the information contained herein is in every respect accurate or complete, and they are not responsible for any errors or omissions or for the results obtained from the use of such information. This is especially true, in particular, when an athlete or person in pain receives Prolotherapy and a bad result occurs. The authors, publishers, and editors of this book do not warrant that Prolotherapy is going to be effective in any medical condition and cannot guarantee or endorse any certain type of Prolotherapy, solution used, or practitioner. It is the responsibility of the individual athlete or person who receives Prolotherapy to thoroughly research the topic and pick a particular practitioner that they feel is qualified to perform the procedure. As of this writing there is no certification available in Prolotherapy training. Any licensed medical or osteopathic doctor in the United States can perform Prolotherapy according to the laws.

Physicians should use and apply the technique of Prolotherapy only after they have received extensive training and demonstrated the ability to safely administer the treatment. The author, publisher, editors, or any other person involved in this work, is not responsible if physicians who are unqualified in the use of Prolotherapy administer the treatment based solely on the contents of this book, or if they receive training but do not administer it safely and a bad result occurs.

If Prolotherapy or any other treatment regime described in this book appears to apply to your condition, the authors, publisher, and editors recommend that a formal evaluation be performed by a physician who is competent in treating pain and athletic injuries with Prolotherapy. Those desiring treatment should make medical decisions with the aid of a personal physician. No medical decisions should be made solely on the contents or recommendations made in this book. ■

You always wonder...what if Mickey Mantle's knees didn't give out so early in his career—what records would he have set? How many Super Bowls would Joe Namath have won if his knees were not so severely damaged? How many more Stanley Cups would Bobby Orr have lifted over his head? Wouldn't he have been the greatest hockey player of all time if he hadn't had such bad knees?

These athletes played in another era when surgical procedures to repair damaged knees were not as sophisticated as those of today. *But*—what about today's athletes who have had the benefit of the latest in medical surgical science, anti-inflammatories and pain killers? Aren't there still many athletes, famous and not, who have had to give up careers because of knee injuries?

This book is dedicated to those athletes who have been told, "surgery will no longer be a benefit," "your career is over," and, "arthritis and eventual knee replacement is what you have to look forward to."

We dedicate this book to you because Prolotherapy is about *another* chance to play. Do you find yourself in this list?

- *The athletes who know that getting arthroscopy is not going to solve their knee problems.*
- *Parents who won't let their young athletes take anti-inflammatory medications.*
- *Chronic knee pain sufferers who are surfing the net because their doctors have no answers.*
- *People who are furious because their years of cortisone shots left them with a degenerated knee, but are still hopeful for an answer to their pain.*
- *Those who are elderly who refuse to go from a cane to a wheelchair because of bad knees.*
- *The average joe who loves his/her sport and will find a way to get rid of their pain so they can continue to play.*
- *The elite athlete who will continue to exercise and play their sport because there has to be answer to their chronic knee problems*
- *The physician who knows deep in his or her heart that no pain is due to an ibuprofen deficiency.*
- *The Prolotherapists out there who continue to help those suffering with chronic pain, despite what the orthopedists say.*

If you are an athlete, or simply a person wishing to remain active, be encouraged! The chronic pain and sports medicine world will be turned upside-down through the first line of treatment we offer you here—Prolotherapy.

This book is also dedicated to the person that gave my wife Marion and I the courage to write and self publish our first book on Prolotherapy, *Prolo Your Pain Away!*, Barry Weiner. Barry said "Ross you have to write a book on Prolotherapy and the injured knee." Barry, you are the best. What my wife says, I sometimes do. What you say I do. I hope you like this book! ■

by Gregg Hill

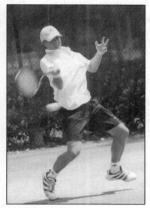

Gregg Hill has been playing tennis since the tender age of five and his professional career began in 1996. He attended the University of Southern California and played tennis there for one year. Gregg was plagued with injuries and didn't think he'd ever play competitive tennis again until he discovered Dr. Hauser and Prolotherapy in February of 1997. Four weeks later, he was back on the courts! Gregg has been a member of the ATP tour for many years, and looks forward to many more years of competitive tennis thanks to Prolotherapy!

Gregg Hill

HOW PROLOTHERAPY SAVED MY GAME

In 1994 all eyes were on Gregg Hill. I was the big story on 60 Minutes that year. Tennis had been my life since I was 10 years old and all the hard work was finally paying off. I was going to be the next big tennis star.

The following year the prediction seemed to be coming true. I was ranked number one junior doubles player in the world and I beat the best junior singles players in the world. But it was at the end of 1995 when I started to have trouble with my right wrist. I had never had any injuries in my life, so the only way I knew how to deal with it was just to play through the pain. I didn't tell anybody. I just kept playing.

In 1996, I went pro and that's when my wrist really began to hurt. I couldn't even play video games; I'd just touch the buttons a few times and my right wrist would start to swell up. Although I was right-handed, before tournaments I would play with my left hand, to save my sore wrist, and then when I went to the tournament I would grip the racket normally and play. I did this throughout 1996 until I finally got to the point where I just couldn't play anymore. The pain was excruciating.

During the year, I had been given two cortisone shots. But they didn't seem to do much good. So, on the recommendation of another professional tennis player, I went to see a surgeon in California. I hadn't looked into surgery before because previous x-rays and MRIs hadn't shown anything. Other doctors had told me my wrist pain was just a sprain. But I had had sprains before and I knew that this pain was different.

When the surgeon in California looked at the x-rays he found that I had a partial tear of a ligament and also a major cyst in my wrist. He told me he could fix my injury with surgery. Finally someone knew how to help my wrist! I was relieved. He said that within a month and a half I'd be playing again. That sounded pretty good to me. I thought, what's a month and a half?

After the surgery, I was told that the injury was fixed. No problem. The surgeon told me to go back home and in a month and a half I'd be ready to play. A month and a half came and went, but my wrist didn't improve. In fact, it hurt just as much as before. The pain was horrible. It felt as if my hand was broken. I kept trying things, like acupuncture. I had never had an injury in my life. I felt so helpless. Everything was new to me, and I was freaking out.

It took about seven months before I finally stumbled across Dr. Hauser on the Internet. His website said that he helped people with terrible pain using a treatment I had never heard of called Prolotherapy. At the time, I didn't think it could help me, but I decided to call him anyway. I knew playing tennis was over for me. I had already had another cortisone shot—that was three cortisone shots, a surgery, and now another new doctor wanted to do surgery on me again. I just knew it wasn't right, that surgery wasn't going to do anything. I had no faith. So I called Dr. Hauser instead.

I could tell on the phone that he was really busy; but I was persistent and I didn't let him get off the phone. I told him, "Listen to me, I'm a professional athlete. I need you to help me." He asked how soon I could get to Chicago. Although I was in Florida, I told him, "I'll see you tomorrow." So I got a plane flight and was there the next day.

I had read that Prolotherapy had a ninety-five percent success rate. I had no clue what it was, maybe a machine they hooked me up to. I thought, we'll see, but I'm sure he can't fix me. Not with my luck. But after meeting Dr. Hauser and talking to him about what was going to happen, my outlook began to change. The moment he gave me the first Prolotherapy injection, I had this incredible peace. I just knew it was going to work.

I received Prolotherapy on my wrist six times—every Friday for six weeks. The treatments eased the pain immediately, but it was about three weeks after the first treatment that my wrist started feeling really strong, and it kept getting stronger. It was like a domino effect, with each treatment helping the others and causing more and more ligament healing and cartilage growth. I started playing four weeks after my first treatment and within three or four days I was hitting backhands with that wrist almost as hard I could. In fact, today my right wrist is stronger than my left. I haven't had a treatment on that wrist in four years.

When I first met Dr. Hauser, I wasn't in the best shape. I had zero energy and was stressed out. We went out to lunch one day and I ordered a sausage pizza and a large Sprite. He had a salad, but I didn't think anything of it at the time. Later he talked to me about my diet and the importance of eating like a champion. He showed me a lot of things I didn't know, like how all the carbohydrates and sugar I was eating had almost made me hypoglycemic, and how that was blocking my healing. He started me on a diet and nutritional supplement program. I had an incredible increase in energy. It's funny, I had gone to a really elite academy that was focused on tennis and conditioning, and I really had no knowledge of injury prevention or nutrition.

About two months after my wrist had healed, I played my first professional tournament. It was incredible, not only to play again, which I was sure would never be possible, but to live and play pain free. Still, it wasn't long before I was plagued with another injury. Falling after hitting a backhand shot, I fractured my elbow and tore some of the ligaments that hold it together; a doctor wanted to do surgery but I said no. It was as though my wrist was the starting point for a series of breakdowns, after all the years of wear and tear. The elbow fracture healed on its own and Prolotherapy promoted healing of the ligaments in that area. I now understood that surgery was not the answer.

Later, I went back to Dr. Hauser again for a partial ACL tear. In fact, to this day, if I don't get Prolotherapy on my shoulder every so often, I can't play. I also know that there are certain injuries that Prolotherapy alone can't help, like my ripped rotator cuff from impingement syndrome. If I had just gone and gotten Prolotherapy, the tear would still be there. But when it comes to pretty much anything else, I go to Dr. Hauser. I don't even go to an orthopedist.

Over the years, I've bought all of Dr. Hauser's books and have read every inch of them. Recently, I was supposed to appear on a talk show with Dr. Hauser but his flight was cancelled, so I had to do it by myself with a group of doctors. It ran on television just about every week for a year and it was funny to watch because I really knew what I was talking about. Before my injury, I didn't know anything. I had never even heard of cortisone. I was really lost when it came to medicine, which was probably a good thing because it made me more open to trying Prolotherapy.

My career is back in full force, now. I'm on tour and doing really well. Next year is going to be a big year for me. Because of all that happened, I'm peaking a little later than I should, but it's better than not playing at all. There's no opportunity to rest in this sport and, for most people, injuries like the ones I had would end their career. Prolotherapy isn't common knowledge and it's not on the TV everyday, and because of that some people want nothing to do with it. I had cortisone shots and they didn't do any good. I had surgery and it was a traumatic experience, and it didn't address my pain at all. But these procedures are routine in the world. Prolotherapy, on the other hand, is simple, has no real side effects, and only takes about three minutes. But the real difference is that it works. The truth is, if it wasn't for Prolotherapy, I wouldn't be playing tennis today. ■

Gregg Hill

Our (my wife and I) first book, *Prolo Your Pain Away! Curing Chronic Pain with Prolotherapy* was released in October of 1997. We were not quite prepared for the response we received to our book. We not only sold all of our printed copies, but we were inundated with calls from chronic pain sufferers, as well as physicians wanting to learn more about this technique of Prolotherapy. This is what we had hoped to accomplish with the book: to make chronic pain sufferers aware of a curative technique that can help end their suffering.

The response to our second book, *Prolo Your Sports Injuries Away! Curing Sports Injuries and Enhancing Athletic Performance with Prolotherapy* has been even more overwhelming. The first book explained a new and different option for chronic pain sufferers: Prolotherapy. The chronic pain community was rattled a bit because of this. However, when you read the chapter in *Prolo Your Sports Injuries Away!* entitled, "The Twenty Myths of Sports Injuries" you will understand why the sports medicine industry was and is still shaking.

For some, the task of reading the 900-plus page *Prolo Your Sports Injuries Away!* is too daunting a task. For these people, I have written this book, *Prolotherapy: An Alternative to Knee Surgery*. The most common cause for arthroscopy or a total joint replacement is an injured knee. The most common cause for lack of mobility in an elderly person—is an injured knee. It's about time for a book to be written telling folks about the healing power of Prolotherapy for the injured knee.

WHAT IS PROLOTHERAPY?

The primary concept that must be understood here is that the fundamental process by which the human body heals and strengthens is inflammation. The traditional philosophy of using some type of anti-inflammatory method such as rest, ice, elevation, compression, anti-inflammatory medications, or cortisone shots to heal injury is totally flawed. No inflammation, no healing. It is that simple.

The concept of Prolotherapy is radical compared to traditional treatments for chronic pain and sports injuries, yet it is so simple. Inject a mild irritant or proliferant at the site of the pain or injury to stimulate healing to the specific area. This concept is too basic for the highly intellectual scholars in the field of chronic pain management. Healing the multitude of chronic painful conditions with such a technique is unthinkable.

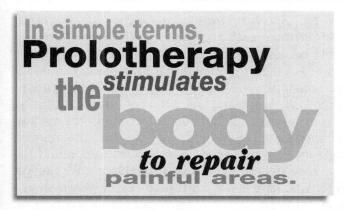

In simple terms, **Prolotherapy** the *stimulates* **body** *to repair* painful areas.

Prolotherapy as defined by *Webster's Third New International Dictionary,* is "the rehabilitation of an incompetent structure, such as a ligament or tendon, by the induced proliferation of cells." "Prolo" comes from the word proliferate (or grow). Prolotherapy injections proliferate or stimulate the growth of new, normal ligament and tendon tissue.

Prolotherapy is based on the concept that the cause of most chronic musculoskeletal pain is ligament and/or tendon weakness (or laxity). Ligaments connect the bones together to provide stability for the joints whereas; tendons connect muscles to the bone providing movement of the joints. When ligaments become weakened, the overlying muscles contract to stabilize the particular joints because the ligaments can no longer do their job. The result is muscle spasms and "knots." Movement is painful because the tendons are weakened and the muscles are spasming. Stimulating the growth with Prolotherapy, thereby strengthening the ligaments and tendons, can relieve most chronic painful conditions.

In simple terms, Prolotherapy stimulates the body to repair painful areas. This is a good way to explain it to your friends, physicians, family, coaches, or trainers. The painful area is commonly a ligament(s) or tendon(s). Prolotherapy stimulates the body to repair this area. It does this by starting the normal healing mechanisms of the body. The injured athlete or chronic pain patient forms normal, healthy, strong tissue in the painful area after Prolotherapy has been administered, ridding the body of the abnormal, weak, painful tissue.

CONDITIONS TREATED WITH PROLOTHERAPY

When people read *Prolo Your Pain Away! Curing Chronic Pain with Prolotherapy,* they were amazed to find out the number of conditions that Prolotherapy could help. Often a person bought the book just to read the section about headaches or low back pain. They were unaware that Prolotherapy had been successful in eliminating many other painful conditions, such as the pain of arthritis, Fibromyalgia, herniated discs, degenerated discs, spondylolisthesis, migraines, RSD, TMJ, sciatica, tension headaches, osteoporosis, vulvodynia, coccydynia, loose joints, carpal tunnel syndrome, Morton's neuroma, myofascial pain, pregnancy back pain, cancer bone pain, and a host of other painful conditions.

When athletes read *Prolo Your Sports Injuries Away! Curing Sports Injuries and Enhancing Athletic Performance with Prolotherapy,* the same response was seen. Prolotherapy could be done on any ligament or joint of the body. Athletes began passing the word to their teammates that Prolotherapy could be used for ligament sprains, tendonitis, heel spurs, Osgood-Schlatter disease, loose joints, rotator cuff problems, ACL tears, and a host of other joint problems. The book discusses over twenty different sports explaining the typical injuries seen in the various sports and how Prolotherapy can cure the injuries and enhance athletic performance for each sport. Athletes who were told their careers were over went on to have stellar careers after Prolotherapy. We cannot tell you the number of people who have avoided arthroscopes, cortisone shots, another Motrin prescription, meniscal surgery, laminectomies, and a host of other surgical procedures because of these two books.

WHY WRITE THIS BOOK?

People who come to the doctor with unresolved knee pain essentially all give the history of one or more of the following:

- *Use of the RICE treatment after the injury*
- *Anti-inflammatory use*
- *Cortisone Shots*
- *Arthroscopy*
- *Knee Surgery*
- *Total Knee Replacement*

The above is the standard of care for knee pain. All of these have the following in common:

- *They do nothing to repair the underlying physiology which led to the pain in the first place.*
- *They are anti-healing.*
- *The normal inflammatory healing reaction is inhibited.*
- *Promote weakening of the normal joint structures.*
- *They accelerate the degenerative process.*

We all know people whose happiness has been hampered significantly by knee pain. This includes the promising athlete who had his/her career cut short because of a knee injury that wouldn't heal; or the "weekend" warrior who no longer can pound it out with his friends on the handball court; to the grandma, who no longer goes shopping with her daughter and grandkids because of immobility. Because of these people this book had to be written.

It is time to change the system. This book is just another step to help people realize that the body heals by inflammation. When a person gets an injury to a joint, the inflammatory process must be stimulated not inhibited. If the injury does not heal, then a specific stimulus to the site of pain and injury must be given for maximum healing to take place. This book is about that stimulus—Prolotherapy. ■

[signature]

Ross Hauser, M.D.

CHAPTER 1

Why Your Knee Didn't Heal

O ver one million Americans this year will have knee surgery. More than five hundred thousand of these will be arthroscopies and two hundred and fifty thousand will be total knee replacements. Most of these orthopedic surgeries will be done in an attempt to relieve the pain of a degenerated knee. How come there are so many degenerated knees?

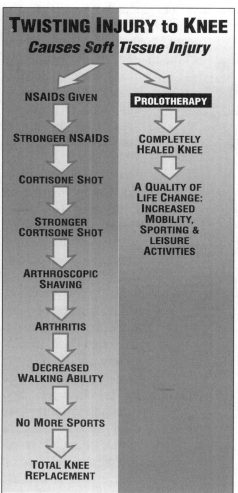

TWISTING INJURY to KNEE
Causes Soft Tissue Injury

NSAIDs GIVEN

PROLOTHERAPY

STRONGER NSAIDS

COMPLETELY
HEALED KNEE

CORTISONE SHOT

A QUALITY OF
LIFE CHANGE:
INCREASED
MOBILITY,
SPORTING &
LEISURE
ACTIVITIES

STRONGER
CORTISONE SHOT

ARTHROSCOPIC
SHAVING

ARTHRITIS

DECREASED
WALKING ABILITY

NO MORE SPORTS

TOTAL KNEE
REPLACEMENT

Figure 1-1: Traditional Orthopedic Care vs. Prolotherapy
One path leads to a total knee replacement. The other leads to a totally normal knee—which would you rather have?

The history in most folks, including elite athletes, is that they had a simple soft tissue injury, either a strain or a sprain. An injury to a tendon or muscle is called a strain, whereas an injury to a ligament is called a sprain. After the injury, the coach, athletic trainer, or physician prescribes the **R.I.C.E.** protocol. This includes rest, ice, compression, and elevation of the leg. Because the injury didn't heal, a nonsteroidal anti-inflammatory medicine Then the infamous cortisone shot is stuck right into the area of pain. Many people get two or three of these. What most people don't realize is that to this point everything that was done promoted *non-healing* of the injury. You see all of these treatments are anti-inflammatories which inhibit the normal healing reaction of the body which is inflammatory. Eventually the cartilage decays because of the above scenario and arthroscopy is done to "clean out" the joint. Generally by this time, the person can no longer run because of the pain, thus, no more sports. Given enough time then a total knee replacement. So in this case, the person had two orthopedic surgeries. A much simpler approach is to get Prolotherapy. *(See Figure 1-1.)*

People reading this book are either looking for alternatives to help heal their injured knee or have already experienced the "knife treatment" (surgery) and still need their injured knee healed. The first step in healing an injured knee is to *stimulate inflammation because inflammation is how the body heals*. Any treatments given that decrease the normal inflammatory healing reaction will decrease the body's chances to heal the injured area.

Imagine a person strains their knee and starts having pain. In simplistic term the pain is a signal to the patient and the physician that something is weakened in the joint. To get rid of the pain the structure must be strengthened. In the knee there are ten main structures that can be injured *(See Figures 1-2, 1-3, 1-4.)*

In the list are five ligaments, two menisci, one articular cartilage, one group of tendons (pes anserinus) and only one muscle (quadriceps). The main difference between muscles and the rest of the structures is that muscles are massively strong structures with a tremendous blood supply, both outside and inside the muscle (this is why steak is red). Ligaments (representatives of all the rest of the structures), on the other hand, are small tissues that have a poor blood supply (why they appear white). *(See Figure 1-5.)* Muscles, because of their good circulation, heal quickly and rarely cause a long-term problem, whereas ligaments, due to their poor blood supply, often heal incompletely and are the cause of most chronic sports injuries and resultant chronic knee pain. The reason that most elite and joe recreational athletes give up their sports is because of nonhealing ligament injuries of the knee.

There are ten main structures that can be injured to cause chronic knee pain. Many of them are seen in this anterior view of the knee.

Articular facet for patella
Medial condyle
Posterior cruciate ligament
Tibial collateral ligament
Medial meniscus
Transverse ligament
Deep infrapatella bursa
Patella ligament
Patella
Anterior cruciate ligament
Fibular collateral ligament
Lateral meniscus
Fibular head
Aperture for blood vessels
Interosseous membrane

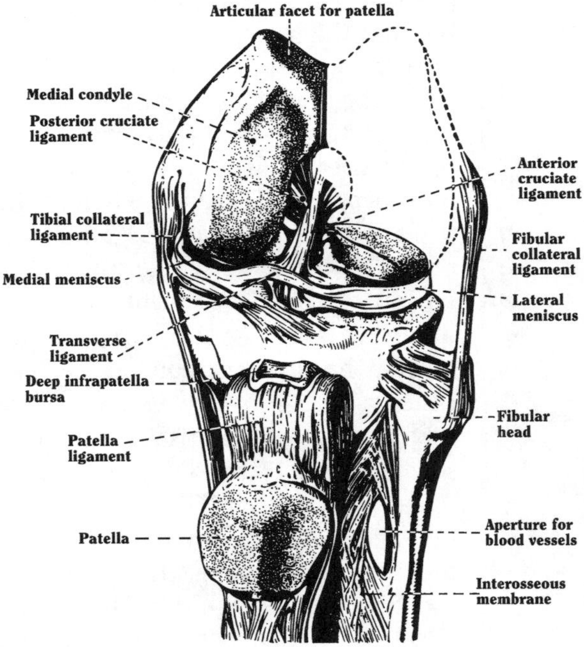

Figure 1-2: Anterior View of the Knee
The large cruciate ligaments inside the knee are the main stabilizers of the knee. Injury to these ligaments puts a tremendous strain on the remaining knee structures and accelerates the degenerative process.

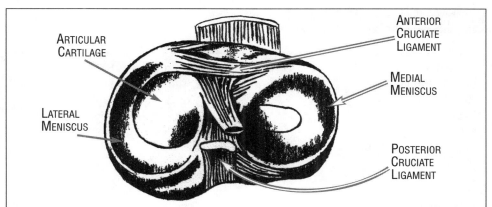

Figure 1-3: Knee Joint From Above From this view it is easy to see the articular cartilage, menisci, and cruciate ligament attachments. These are common areas that are torn or weakened in the injured knee.

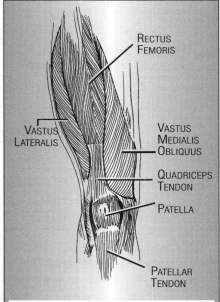

Figure 1-4: Knee Joint Muscle Attachments

The quadriceps muscle attachments are common structures injured causing knee pain.

R.I.C.E. Is Not So Nice

The **R.I.C.E.** treatment is the gold standard for pain management and sports injuries today. Just go to any emergency room or sports trainer with an acute knee sprain or other joint injury, and the injured person will be given these instructions: **R**est, **I**ce, **C**ompression and **E**levation. Most people would also receive instructions to take anti-inflammatory medications. This treatment is recommended because ligament sprains, that is, meniscal /articular cartilage injuries, are often accompanied by quite a bit of swelling, called edema. The premise with the **R.I.C.E.** treatment is that the swelling and edema is harmful to the tissue.

Understanding the difference between muscles and rest of the structures around the knee is crucial to understanding why the **R.I.C.E.** treatment is totally inappropriate for healing ligaments, menisci, tendons, and articular cartilage injuries. Muscles, such as the quadriceps, occupy an entire thigh, and have the strength and power to allow some athletes, like weight lifters, to squat in excess of 800 pounds. Muscles are the structures that move the joints. Contrast this to most ligaments, which are generally less than one inch in length, and whose width is measured in millimeters. These small structures have the job of binding the bones together. The menisci and

COMPARISON OF MUSCLES AND LIGAMENTS

	MUSCLES	LIGAMENTS
Function	Movement	Stability
Circulation by	Large arteries	Small arterioles
Blood supply	Excellent	Poor
Repair ability	Excellent	Poor
Chronic injuries	Rare	High
Appearance (based on blood supply)	Red	White
Size	Feet	Millimeters
Location in relationship to the joints (in general)	Outside	Inside
Insertion site	Tendons	Bone
Compartments	Fascial	None
Stretch ability	Good	Poor
Injury severity	Mild	Moderate
Response to exercise	Dramatic	Little

Figure 1-5: Muscles are massively strong structures with a tremendous blood supply. Ligaments, on the other hand, are small tissues with a poor blood supply.

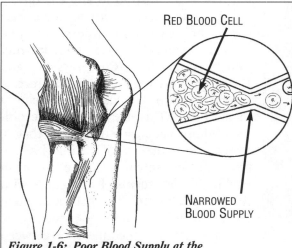

RED BLOOD CELL

NARROWED BLOOD SUPPLY

Figure 1-6: Poor Blood Supply at the Fibro-Osseous Junction
The fibro-osseous junction of ligaments normally has a poor blood supply compared to other structures such as muscles.

articular likewise, have their widths measured in millimetes and have the important task of cushioning the joints, as in the knee.

Muscles have a tremendous arterial blood supply, that can increase 25-fold during strenuous exercise. Ligaments, articular cartilage, menisci, and many tendons have terrible blood supplies. The menisci and articular cartilage depend on the joint fluid for their nutrition. The ligaments normally receive blood vessels from small arterial plexuses from the joints, but they themselves have essentially no blood vessels. This implies that at least some degree of their nutrition must come from diffusion of nutrients, most likely from the joint itself. Much like the articular cartilage and menisci. The actual insertion sites of ligaments into bones, called the fibro-osseous junction, are also essentially avascular (without blood supply). It should be evident now why ligaments are so easily injured. A joint is jostled during an athletic event. The small blood vessels to the joint are sheared. The little blood supply that the ligaments had is then cut off. The body has to repair the damage, but how can it do so if no immune cells can get to the area because of the poor blood supply? The blood supply to the ligaments is the worst at the point where the ligament attaches to the bone, called the fibro-osseous junction. *(See Figure 1-6.)* This is the weak link in the ligament-bone complex. This is the most common area injured in the athlete and is responsible for much of the chronic knee pain that people feel. This is the exact site where Prolotherapy is administered.

As a result of immobilization (rest), ice, compression, and elevation blood flow is decreased to the knee or joint where it is used, resulting in reduced immune cell production necessary to remove the debris from the injury site. This produces formation of weak ligament and tendon tissue. The ligament-bone interface is tremendously susceptible to the effects of immobility or disuse. *(See Figure 1-7.)* For instance in one study, just nine weeks in plaster cast caused the medical collateral ligament to lose 39 percent of its strength due to bone resorption at the point where the ligament attaches to the bone. Although muscle weight returned to normal by around 12 weeks, bone remineralization was not complete at 24 weeks and ligament strength was still not normal at 30 weeks. This is another reason why you cannot treat muscle injuries the same way you treat ligament injuries. They are microscopically, anatomically, physiologically different than ligaments. Ligaments, like menisci and articular cartilage, are tremendously sensitive to the detrimental effects of rest, immobilization, ice, anti-inflammatories, and cortisone shots. For these reasons, athletes and others who want to heal must say "no" to these therapies.

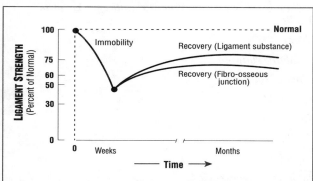

Figure 1-7: Detrimental Effects of Immobility on Ligament Strength
Recovery or strength of the bone-ligament (fibro-osseous) junction occurs much slower than the ligament substance itself. Both bone and ligaments often do not completely heal.

Swelling after an injury is the physical manifestation of inflammation. Swelling is evidence that the body is working to heal itself. Use of ice (and the **R.I.C.E.** protocol) will obviously prevent the body from repairing the injury. It has been shown that as little as five minutes of icing a knee can decrease both blood flow to the soft tissues and skeletal metabolism. Icing an area for 25 minutes, which is what most people and athletic trainers do, decreases blood flow to the soft tissues and skeletal metabolism by 400 percent. Healing is thus hindered by a decrease in blood flow and metabolism to the area. Icing (and the **R.I.C.E.** protocol) increases the chance of incomplete healing by decreasing blood flow to the injured ligaments, tendons, menisci, and cartilage. This increases the chance of re-injury or the development of chronic pain.

ANTI-INFLAME IS NOT THE WAY

NSAIDs are non-steroidal anti-inflammatory drugs. These are drugs that are not steroids, but their main function to reduce inflammation (just like steroids). NSAIDs are used widely in sports injuries in order to reduce the inflammation which occurs at the site of the injury. Almost anyone with pain that goes to a health care provider will be given an NSAID to relieve them of their pain.

The all-star list of the latest NSAIDs is as follows:

- *Proprionic acid derivatives: Ibuprofen, Naproxen, Anaprox, Sulindac, Daypro, Fenoprofen, Ketoprofen, Orudis*
- *Piroxicams: Piroxicam, Feldene*
- *Phenylacetic: Arthrotec, Cataflam, Voltaren*
- *Indoles: Indomethacin, Sulindac, Tolmetin*
- *Fenamates: Ponstel, Meclofenamate*
- *Salicylates: Aspirin, Ecotrin*
- *Carboxylic acids: Dolobid, Lodine*
- *Others: Relafen, Tolectin, Toradol*
- *The latest stars, COX-2 inhibitors: Celebrex, Vioxx*

A statement taken from a well-known sports medicine book that has gone through five printings is **"In spite of the widespread use of NSAIDs, there is no convincing evidence as to their effectiveness in the treatment of acute soft tissue injuries."** This statement is true, but definitely not strong enough. A more appropriate statement would be something like, "In spite of the widespread use of NSAIDs, there is substantial evidence that they hamper ligament, tendon, menisci, and articular cartilage healing. Using them will surely delay and possibly even prevent an injury from healing."

In 1993 at the University of North Carolina School of Medicine, Division of Orthopaedic Surgery, Sports Medicine section, Dr. Louis Almekinders and associates performed a study on human tendon fibroblasts to measure the effects of exercise and the NSAID Indomethacin on the fibroblasts. Fibroblasts are the cells that actually grow the collagen that makes up ligaments, tendons, and menisci tissue.

The Study Groups Were as Follows:

- **Group 1:** *The control in which no treatment was done.*
- **Group 2:** *The tendons were exercised.*

- **Group 3:** *The tendons were exercised and anti-inflamed with the NSAID Indomethacin.*
- **Group 4:** *The tendons were just anti-inflamed with the Indomethacin.*

All the tendons underwent injury through repetitive motion, similar to what would happen to an athlete in training. At 72 hours after the injury, it was noted that compared to controls the only group that had increased levels of prostaglandins was the exercised group. The group that was exercised and received the NSAID, as well as the NSAID group, had statistically significantly lower levels of prostaglandins (specifically Prostaglandin E2, a normal component of the inflammatory cascade) in the tendons. This showed that the NSAID blocked the inflammatory healing of even the tendon injuries that were exercised or rehabilitated. The tendonitis that was treated with just the NSAID had almost no prostaglandins in the sample, signaling a complete inhibition of the inflammatory healing process. The effect was even more pronounced at 108 hours. *(See Figure 1-8.)*

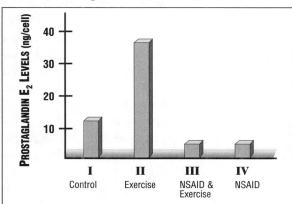

Figure 1-8: Levels of Prostaglandin E2 in the Medium Around Tendon Fibroblasts
Group II exercise-treated tendons, show an enhanced inflammatory response, compared to Control Group I. The groups receiving NSAIDs (III and IV) showed no healing inflammatory response at all.

The researchers also measured DNA synthesis in the fibroblasts, with the level increasing if the cells were proliferating. Again the exercised group was the only group with elevated levels of DNA synthesis in the fibroblasts. Compared to the control group there was 100 percent more growth of fibroblasts. The tendons treated with Indomethacin had no DNA synthesis noted. *(See Figure 1-9.)* This showed there was no fibroblastic growth occurring. The group that exercised and took the NSAID showed a little bit of growth. The authors concluded, "Motion and prostaglandin release in Group 2 were associated with increased DNA synthesis. Inhibition of prostaglandin by indomethacin also coincided with a decrease in DNA synthesis... Inhibition of prostaglandin synthesis, and thereby DNA synthesis, may not be desirable during the proliferative stage of a soft tissue injury, when DNA synthesis for cell division of fibroblasts is needed to heal the injury to the tendon."[1] The paper also stated a fact that many researchers in this field are wondering, "Despite the lack of scientific data, NSAIDs are widely used, often as the mainstay of treatment."

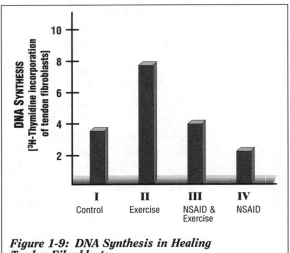

Figure 1-9: DNA Synthesis in Healing Tendon Fibroblasts

DNA synthesis in the fibroblasts is clearly stimulated by exercise and inhibited by NSAIDs.

In another study on the use of perhaps the most popular anti-inflammatory drug used in sports medicine, ibuprofen, in the treatment of tendon injuries, it was found that the ibuprofen used in the study decreased the strength of the flexor tendons undergoing repair by 300 percent at four weeks. The peak force of the flexor tendons of controls was 12.0 newtons, whereas in the Indomethacin group it was an average of 2.5 newtons. Extensor tendon analysis showed similar results with controls having a breaking strength of 12.0 newtons and the tendons treated with the NSAID 3.5 newtons. The authors noted, "Examination of the data reveals a marked decrease in the breaking strength of tendons at four and six weeks in the ibuprofen-treated animals... This difference was statistically significant." [2]

These last two studies should make any athlete who has suffered a sports injury, only to have it treated with ibuprofen or any other NSAID, shudder. Yes, you may not now have pain, but you sure do not have strength. Athletes, you need to repair the area when it is injured by proliferating brand new ligament and tendon tissue. The best way to do this is using **MEAT** treatments, followed by Prolotherapy (explained in the next chapter).

Ligaments and tendons consist mainly of collagen. One study found that up to 99 percent of the tendon by dry weight is collagen.[3] The mechanical stability of collagen is thus the most important factor for the mechanical strength of the tissue. Furthermore, since fibroblasts make collagen, fibroblastic growth is therefore crucial to ligament and tendon growth. From the above studies, it is clear that NSAIDs inhibit the fibroblastic growth process and thus diminish an athlete's chance of healing.

NSAIDs are used because they decrease pain, but they do so at the expense of hurting the healing of the injured soft tissue. A good example of this is a study on the use of Piroxicam (NSAID) in the treatment of acute ankle sprains in the Australian military. Compared with the placebo group, the subjects treated with Piroxicam had less pain, were able to resume training more rapidly, were treated at lower cost, and were found to have increased exercise endurance on resumption of activity. The conclusion of the study was that NSAIDs should form an integral part of the treatment of acute ankle sprains. At first glance in reviewing this study, NSAIDs appear to be a great thing. The real question is did they help the ligament injury heal? In reviewing the study the answer is a resounding "no."

To test ligament healing, the ankles were tested via the anterior drawer test. During this test the ankle was moved forward to see how much laxity there was in the ligaments. This study was published in 1997 and the author stated that this was the first time the clinical measurement of the anterior drawer sign had been used in a clinical trial. It meant that all the studies done prior to this one in assessing whether anti-inflammatories helped with ankle sprains did not test whether the ligaments healed or not. In this study, at every date of testing after the initial injury, days three, seven, and 14, the Piroxicam-treated group demonstrated greater ligament instability. At the time of the initial injury, the ligament instability in the Piroxicam group and the control group were exactly the same. This study showed that the NSAID use stopped ligament healing, yet the subjects felt better. The authors noted, "This result is of concern in that it may reflect a paradoxically adverse effect of the NSAID-derived analgesia in allowing subjects to resume activity prematurely." [4]

Do you see the difference between pain relief and healing? The athlete or pain patient needs to heal the tissue. Up until the present, when it came to ligament injuries, too many studies were advocating NSAID use because they were such great pain-relievers, when in fact they were and are stopping the healing mechanisms of the body. Any technique or medication that stops the normal inflammatory process that helps heal the body must have a long-term detrimental effect on the body. Nothing shows this more clearly than the use of steroids in both sports injuries and chronic pain management.

STANDARD OF CARE
REVIEW OF THE RESEARCH ON NSAIDS AND CORTICOSTEROIDS

Cortisone shots are still considered the standard of care for the injured athlete. The leading article just a few years ago in *Sports Medicine* advocated the treatment regime as depicted in *Figure 1-10.*

NSAIDs

You can see that NSAIDs were recommended for the first three to five days and steroid injections were recommended within the first 24 hours. [5] According to the article, both treatments should be done because they decreased inflammation. The texts *Essentials of Musculoskeletal Care* published by both the American Academy of Orthopedic Surgeons (the main organization for orthopaedic surgeons) and the American Academy of Pediatrics (the main one for pediatricians) states, "Inflammation is an essential, normal protective mechanism associated with injury to the musculoskeletal system. The pain associated with inflammation is the "gift that nobody wants." [6] It then goes on to say how NSAIDs are used to treat such conditions as tendonitis. The problem with this advice is that it is totally contradictory. On the one hand, the main groups of Orthopaedic

SUMMARY OF MODES OF TREATMENT FOR ACUTE MUSCULAR INJURIES

Mode of Treatment	When Treated	Effect
Rest	24-48 hours in Grade I-II	Decrease swelling Decrease hemorrhage
	3-5 weeks in Grade III unless repaired	Allows bridging of the defect
Ice	24-48 hours	Decrease swelling Slow metabolism Pain control
Compression & elevation	24-48 hours	Decrease swelling
NSAIDs	3-5 days	Pain control Decrease inflammation
Steroid injection	Within 24 hours	Decrease inflammation
Proteolytic enzymes	Within 24 hours	Decrease hematoma
Mobilization	Grades I-II	Prevent contracture Prevent weakness

Figure 1-10:
Today steroid shots and NSAIDs are still considered the standard of care for traumatic and sports injuries.

Surgeons and Pediatricians recently published a text in 1997, saying that inflammation is normal and protective, yet they are advising in the same text to give medications that stop inflammation! Guess what will happen when you wipe out something that is protective? The result is no more protection, and subsequent injury. It has to happen and it will happen!

CORTICOSTEROIDS

The same authors go on to say regarding corticosteroids, "Corticosteroids suppress the initial events in inflammation. They decrease collagenase and prostaglandin formation and formation of granulation tissue. They are catabolic promoters that block glucose uptake in the tissues, enhance protein breakdown, and decrease new protein synthesis in muscle, skin, bone, connective tissue, and lymphoid tissue."[6] There you have it right from the definitive source-the leading body of Orthopaedic surgeons and pediatricians just said, in print, exactly what steroids do! This is, in essence, their confession. First and foremost they suppress the initial effects of inflammation. What happens after the athletic injury? Inflammation. Next they state that corticosteroids stop prostaglandin formation and granulation tissue. In lay terms, the next things suppressed are the mediators that help new tissue formation, the prostaglandins. Prostaglandins help recruit immune cells to the injured area to clean up the damaged tissue and start the repair process. They also help increase circulation to the injured area. This is all wiped out by corticosteroids. These medications stop granulation tissue formation. What does this mean? Granulation tissue is the tissue that needs to be formed to heal the area. In other words, steroid shots stop new tissue from being formed or at least it slows the process down. *(See Figure 1-11.)*

The American Academy of Orthopaedic Surgeons and the American Academy of Pediatrics then give you further insight on how corticosteroids slow the repair process down—steroids are catabolic promoters. Catabolism means "breakdown." Corticosteroids stimulate the breakdown of tissue. Not only do they suppress the healing mechanisms following an injury, they stimulate the breakdown of that tissue as well as any normal tissue in the area.

Remember the statement, "They are catabolic promoters that block glucose uptake in the tissues, enhance protein breakdown, and decrease new protein synthesis in muscle, skin, bone, connective tissue, and lymphoid tissue (predominantly T-cells)."[6] Corticosteroids stimulate the breakdown of tissue by cutting off the food supply (glucose) to tissues and enhancing the breakdown of the protein in the tissues. Remember that muscle, ligament, and tendon tissue is 70 to 90 percent collagen, which is a protein. The orthopedists tell us that the function of corticosteroids is to decrease the formation of collagen in these connective tissues.

In the section on the use of intra-articular injections (injections of cortisone and other steroids) they state, "Injections into ligamentous structures carry the risk of spontaneous rupture of the ligament and are usually quite painful. The Achilles and patellar (knee) tendons should not be injected in the substance of the tendon since pain in these structures usually indicates interstitial tears, which already have reduced their tensile strength."[6] These statements are exactly right. Steroid injections pose a definite risk to the athlete-tendon and ligament rupture. These are quite painful. You will not have a very happy athlete after that either!

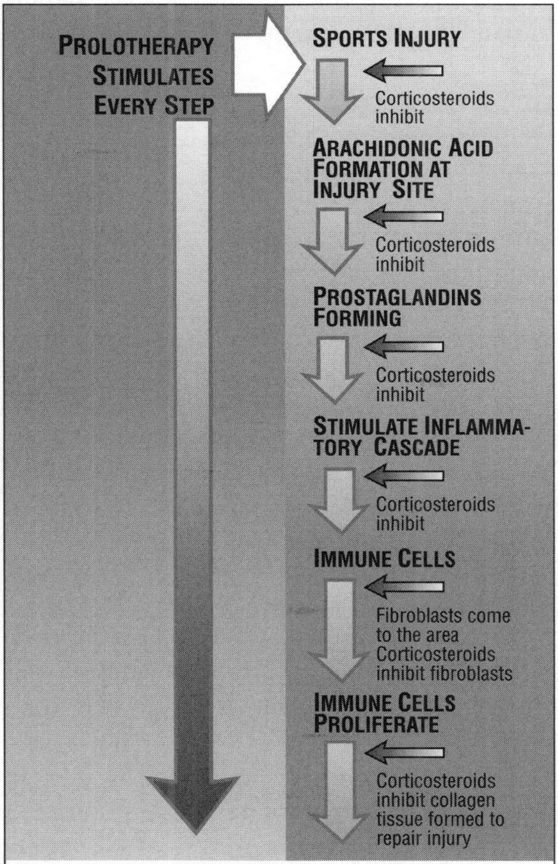

The typical advice in sports medicine is that cortisone injections can be of great value in overuse injuries, such as tendonitis. Such injections should not be given directly into muscles or tendons as they may cause weakening and subsequent rupture of the tissues.[7] They should be given only when specifically indicated and when given, injected only around a muscle or tendon attachment or into the surrounding sheath. Refraining from exercise with load is recommended for two weeks after injection in order to avoid problems.

In other words, they are saying do not inject steroids into the tendons, muscles, or

Figure 1-11: The Healing Inflammatory Cascade
Corticosteroids inhibit every step of the cascade, whereas Prolotherapy injections do the opposite—they enhance it.

PROLOTHERAPY STIMULATES EVERY STEP

SPORTS INJURY
↓ Corticosteroids inhibit

ARACHIDONIC ACID FORMATION AT INJURY SITE
↓ Corticosteroids inhibit

PROSTAGLANDINS FORMING
↓ Corticosteroids inhibit

STIMULATE INFLAMMATORY CASCADE
↓ Corticosteroids inhibit

IMMUNE CELLS
↓ Fibroblasts come to the area Corticosteroids inhibit fibroblasts

IMMUNE CELLS PROLIFERATE
↓ Corticosteroids inhibit collagen tissue formed to repair injury

ligaments, because they could rupture. But injecting around them is okay. This makes no sense whatsoever. To make sure that the soft tissues do not rupture after a steroid injection, don't work out for two weeks? Why? Because the steroid is making your ligaments, tendons, and muscles weaker and we do not want to risk rupture. Athletes and people in pain wake up! Are you paying attention! You guys are receiving shot after shot and put back in the game immediately. You weekend warriors you know the second your knee feels good after a steroid shot, you call your buddy for a handball game, don't you? There is rarely an occasion to give a steroid injection for athletic injuries. Corticosteroids do exactly the opposite of what an athlete is trying to do for the injuries. Athletes work out every day to get stronger, faster, and more skilled at their events. Steroids cause injured tissues to heal poorly and cause the normal tissue to deteriorate. Next time the sports medicine doctor comes with the syringe filled with the milky white stuff ask him/her whether the injection does anything to help the body repair the injured area. The answer must be no, because there is only one type of injection that does that. Prolotherapy.

WHAT IS A CORTICOSTEROID ANYWAY?

Cortisol is the naturally-occurring adrenal gland hormone. There are many synthetic analogues including cortisone (Prednisone), Triamcinolone, Celestone, Dexamethasone, and many others. These synthetic analogues are many times stronger than natural cortisol and are often injected into the athletes' joints, ligaments, and tendons because of their potent anti-inflammatory effects.

Using the main pharmacology text from many medical schools, Goodman and Gilman's *The Pharmacological Basis of Therapeutics*, Seventh Edition, you will see why it is our opinion that cortisone shots have essentially no role in the treatment of athletic injuries. "Cortisol and the synthetic analogs of cortisol have the capacity to prevent or suppress the development of the local heat, redness, swelling, and tenderness by which inflammation is recognized. At the microscopic level, they inhibit not only the early phenomena of the inflammatory process, edema, fibrin deposition, capillary dilatation, migration of leukocytes into the inflamed area, and phagocytic activity, but also the later manifestations of capillary proliferation, fibroblast proliferation, deposition of collagen, and still later cicatrization."[8] Honestly, we do not know what cicatrization is either, but at least we know that corticosteroids inhibit it. (Just kidding! It means healing by scar formation.)

The comparison of cortisone shots to Prolotherapy injections is seen in *Figure 1-12*. Corticosteroids inhibit the inflammatory response no matter whether the inciting agent of the inflammation is trauma from an ankle sprain, knee strain, an infection, or an allergenic food that is eaten. What modern medicine forgets is that steroid therapy is, at best, just palliative therapy—it reduces inflammation and reduces symptoms, but the underlying cause of the disease

FIGURE 1-12: CORTISONE VERSUS PROLOTHERAPY

	CORTISONE	PROLOTHERAPY
Capillary Dilation	Decreased	Increased
Blood Flow	Decreased	Increased
Migration of Immune Cells to Area	Decreased	Increased
Phagocytic Activity (clean up)	Decreased	Increased
Leukocyte Numbers in Area	Decreased	Increased
Capillary Proliferation (new blood vessels)	Decreased	Increased
Fibroblast Proliferation	Decreased	Increased
Deposition of Collagen	Decreased	Increased
Collagen Strength	Decreased	Increased
Protein Synthesis	Decreased	Increased
Tissue Strength	Decreased	Increased

Figure 1-12: Cortisone versus Prolotherapy There really is no comparison.

remains. This is why natural medicine physicians and Prolotherapists use very little cortisone in their practices. Cortisone, Prednisone, Celestone, and the rest of the synthetic analogues do nothing to repair the damaged tissue. They, in fact, damage the tissues themselves by making them weaker.

It is no longer a question of whether corticosteroids weaken the ligaments, tendons, joints, and cartilage into which they are injected, it is just a matter of how much. One study, done just a few years after corticosteroids became available in injectable form (1954), showed that tendon strength was cut in half by the steroids.[9] Because of the definite risk of tendon rupture with steroid injections, many athletes are refusing to get cortisone shots anymore.[10] Numerous other studies have shown that corticosteroids lead to a decrease in bone, ligament, and tendon strength.[11-13] In one astonishing study on corticosteroid injections into tendons, a full 100 percent of the tendons injected had tendon necrosis (death) at the site of the injection.[14] Another study confirmed this, but added the fact that tendon tissue necrosis after steroid injection can be seen in 45 minutes.[15] Yes, you heard us correctly! After 45 minutes, the tendon could be necrosing while the athlete is still in the game.

Under a microscope, tendons injected with cortisone show disruption of the collagen bundles with deposits of steroid in them.[16] The tendon strength in another study was down by 35 percent only two days after a corticosteroid injection. The reduced strength in the tendon was still evident seven days later.[17]

Steroids have the same detrimental effect on ligaments. Many athletes are duped into getting a steroid shot so they can play in a game. Their reasoning, "Ah, it is only one shot. It can't hurt." You better think again. One shot of cortisone has already been shown to decrease the tensile strength of the anterior cruciate ligament of the knee by up to 39 percent when tested one full year after the injection.[18] This study also confirmed that fibroblastic cells were actually **killed** by the corticosteroid injection.

Many studies have documented the inhibitory effects of corticosteroids on collagen formation.[19-22] This leads you to assume that steroids would inhibit ligament healing because ligaments are comprised of 70 to 80 percent collagen by dry weight. This is exactly what study after study has shown.

A recent study at Brown University School of Medicine showed that **only one** corticosteroid injection at day two or day seven after a ligament injury produced long-term detrimental effects. More specifically, the steroid-injected ligaments showed smaller cross sectional areas, lower peak load force, and lower energy to peak load force. *(See Figure 1-13.)* The authors noted, "These results suggest that the properties of the collagenous matrix, histological appearance, and bio-mechanical properties are significantly altered by a one-time steroid injection given immediately following or seven days after injury."[23] Athletes should never assume, "It's just a steroid injection."

To determine the extent of the damage done by steroids, Michael E. Wiggins, M.D., and associates, at Brown University School of Medicine performed two studies on the healing characteristics of ligaments treated with corticosteroids. They first determined the effects of different concentrations of corticosteroids (Betamethasone) on collagen synthesis by the fibroblasts. *Figure 1-14* shows us that the steroid significantly inhibited collagen synthesis.

They next studied the effect of a single steroid shot on ligament healing. A decrease in strength as measured by peak load was determined to be upwards of 50 percent. The authors concluded that a single corticosteroid injection into an acutely injured ligament has "...significant inhibitory effects on the healing process in the early phases (inflammatory, matrix, and cellular proliferation) of ligament healing...with the higher dose steroid (human equivalent dose), almost a **complete inhibition** of healing occurred."[24]

This research won the 1992 Excellence in Research Award from *American Journal of Sports Medicine*. The question therefore remains. If the research is so good and so conclusive, why do athletes continue to receive steroid shots? The authors showed in a follow-

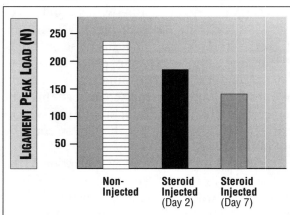

Figure 1-13: Ligament Peak Load Strength at Three Months

One steroid injection into an injured ligament, whether on day two or seven post-injury, caused a significant decline in ligament strength at three months.

Adapted from **Healing Characteristics of a Type I Collagenous Structure Treated with Corticosteroids** *by Michael E. Wiggins, M.D., Paul D. Fadale, M.D., Hans Barrach, M.D., Michael G. Ehrlich, M.D., and William R. Walsh, M.D.*

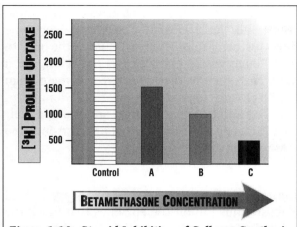

Figure 1-14: Steroid Inhibition of Collagen Synthesis
The [³H] proline uptake as a relative indicator of collagen synthesis of fibroblasts in cell culture when exposed to different concentrations of betamethasone.

Adapted from **Healing Characteristics of a Type I Collagenous Structure Treated with Corticosteroids** *by Michael E. Wiggins, M.D., Paul D. Fadale, M.D., Hans Barrach, M.D., Michael G. Ehrlich, M.D., and William R. Walsh, M.D.*

up study that the effect of the steroids remains even 84 days after the injection. Their conclusion was quite remarkable. "Intensive rehabilitation after injection of corticosteroids around injured type-1 collagenous structures (ligaments and tendons) **could potentially be harmful or lead to a reinjury.**" [25] Listen to what they are saying! If you receive a steroid shot, your ligaments and tendons will get weaker and weaker. If you do a strenuous workout, you may pop your hamstring tendon or cruciate ligament!

As bad as these facts seem, the worst effect of cortisone for athletes is what it does to the cartilage inside the knee where it is commonly injected. As soon as corticosteroids made it into the headlines, by Hench and co-workers, who won the Nobel Prize for medicine for their discovery of them in 1950, physicians were bound and determined to use them anyway they could. It took only one year for The *Journal of the American Medical Association* to report that these new-found steroids could be injected. [26] It didn't take long for physicians to inject, inject, and inject them some more, until reports started coming in that people who received injected steroids into the joints were getting progressive degenerative arthritis. [27] This was because corticosteroids were tremendously detrimental to articular cartilage in the joints. One study showed that even 16 weeks after a **single** joint injection, the cartilage remained biochemically and metabolically impaired. [28]

Steroid injections have been studied in depth. The type of steroid does not matter when it comes to destroying ligament or tendon tissue. It could be a water-soluble or crystalloid "depot" form glucocorticoid. If it is a steroid, it kills cartilage. A study done at University Central Hospital in Helsinki, Finland, confirmed these facts. Significant deleterious effects were seen on cartilage via electron microscopy after only **one** steroid injection into the knee. As expected, the authors found that the more steroid injections that were given into the knee, the worse the deterioration. They concluded, "The deleterious glucocorticoid effects are caused by cartilage digestion of the joint while cartilage elasticity is simultaneously reduced." [29]

Because of all the detrimental effects of corticosteroids, athletes are beginning to wake up and say "no" to cortisone and "yes" to Prolotherapy. While cortisone weakens the damaged athletic injury further, Prolotherapy stimulates the body to repair the injured areas. Athletes are finally wising up to the fact that a long-term cure is much better for them than the quick pain-relief offered to them from steroid injections. For the athlete who chooses to get the steroid shot, a long-term weakened cartilage, ligament, or tendon awaits. Smart athletes are Proloing their sports injuries away because they ultimately want the injured areas stronger so their strength and athletic prowess will remain.

SUMMARY

Local inflammation of the injured ligament or tendon is necessary to heal sports injuries. NSAIDs and corticosteroids inhibit the enzymes that block the production of prostaglandins and leukotrienes, which mediate the inflammatory process. By blocking their production, these medications have a deleterious effect on soft tissue healing by inhibiting blood flow to the injured area, new blood vessel formation, immune cells, like leukocytes and macrophages, from coming to the area, protein synthesis, fibroblast proliferation, and ultimately collagen formation. The collagen that forms in ligaments and tendons treated with NSAIDs and corticosteroids is disrupted and weaker. Because of these effects athletes are starting to refuse these treatments. Prolotherapy has the exact opposite effect. Prolotherapy stimulates blood flow to the area, new blood vessel formation, immune cells to the area, protein synthesis, fibroblast proliferation, and ultimately collagen formation. The end result is that Prolotherapy stimulates the immune system to repair the damaged area. It is for this reason that athletes are saying "no" to the detrimental effects of NSAIDs and cortisone shots and desiring soft tissue repair by Prolotherapy.

For the inquiring mind who wants to research whether this and any other information in this book is true, please check out the complete reference lists in the books *Prolo Your Pain Away!* and *Prolo Your Sports Injuries Away!* ▪

BIBLIOGRAPHY

1. Almekinders, L. An in vitro investigation into the effects of repetitive motion and non-steroidal anti-inflammatory medication on human tendon fibroblasts. *American Journal of Sports Medicine*. 1995; 23:119-123.

2. Kulick, M. Oral ibuprofen: evaluation of its effect on peritendinous adhesions and the breaking strength of a tenorrhaphy. *The Journal of Hand Surgery*. 1986; 11A:110-119.

3. Dale, W. A Composite Materials Analysis of the Structure, Mechanical Properties, and Aging of Collagenous Tissues. *Doctoral Thesis*, Case Western Reserve University, Cleveland, Ohio. 1974.

4. Slatyer, M. A randomized controlled trial of piroxicam in the management of acute ankle sprain in Australian regular army recruits. *American Journal of Sports Medicine*. 1997; 25:544-553.

5. Almekinders, L. Anti-inflammatory treatment of muscular injuries in sports. *Sports Medicine.* 1993; 15:139-145.

6. Snider, R. (editor) Essentials of Musculoskeletal Care. Rosemont, IL: *American Academy of Orthopaedic Surgeons.* 1997, p. 37-48.

7. Peterson, L. Sports Injuries. Chicago, IL: *Year Book Medical Publishers.* 1986, pp. 168-169.

8. Gilman, A. *The Pharmacological Basis of Therapeutics.* Seventh Edition. New York City, NY: Macmillan Publishing Company. 1985, pp. 1463-1485.

9. Wrenn, R. An experimental study of the effect of cortisone on the healing process and tensile strength of tendons. *Journal of Bone and Joint Surgery.* 1954; 36A:588-601.

10. Cyriax, J. *Textbook of Orthopaedic Medicine. Volume One.* London, England: Bailliere Tindall. 1982,p.419.

11. Truhan, A. Corticosteroids: A review with emphasis on complications of prolonged systemic therapy. *Annals of Allergy.* 1989; 62:375-290.

12. Gogia, P. Hydrocortisone and exercise effects on articular cartilage in rats. *Archives of Physical Medicine and Rehabilitation.* 1993; 74:463-467.

13. Chandler, G.N. Deleterious effect of intra-articular hydrocortisone. *Lancet.* 1958; 2:661-663.

14. Ferland, M. Necrose localisee due a une injection intratendineuse de gluco-corticoide: etude experimentale comparative. *Union Med Can.* 1972; 101:1768-1771.

15. Balasubramaniam, P. The effect of injection of hydrocortisone into rabbit calcaneal tendons. *Journal of Bone and Joint Surgery.* 1972; 54:729-734.

16. Unverferth, L. The effect of local steroid injections on tendons. *Journal of Sports Medicine.* 1973; 1:31-37.

17. Kennedy, J. The effects of local steroid injections on tendons: a biomechanical and microscopic correlative study. *American Journal of Sports Medicine.* 1976; 4:11-21.

18. Noyes, F. Biomechanical and ultrastructural changes in ligaments and tendons after local corticosteroid injections. *Journal of Bone and Joint Surgery.* 1975; 57A:876.

19. Anastassiades, T. The effect of cortisone on the metabolism of connective tissues in the rat. *J. Lab Clin Med.* 1970; 75: 826-839.

20. Manthorpe, R. Effects of glucocorticoid on connective tissue of aorta and skin in rabbits. *Acta Endocrinol.* 1974; 77: 310-324.

21. McCoy, B. In vitro inhibition of cell growth, collagen synthesis, and prolyl hydroxylase activity by triamcinolone acetonide. *Proc Soc Exp Biol Med.* 1980; 163: 216-222.

22. Oikarinen, A. Modulation of collagen metabolism by glucocorticoids. *Biochem Pharmacol.* 1988; 37:1451-1462.

23. Walsh, W. Effects of a delayed steroid injection on ligament healing using a rabbit medial collateral ligament model. *Biomaterials.* 1995; 16:905-910.

24. Wiggins, M. Healing characteristics of a type-1 collagenous structure treated with corticosteroids. *American Journal of Sports Medicine.* 1994; 22:279-288.

25. Wiggins, M. Effects of local injection of corticosteroids on the healing of ligaments. *Journal of Bone and Joint Surgery.* 1995; 77A:1682-1691.

26. Hollander, J. Hydrocortisone and cortisone injected into arthritic joints. *Journal of the American Medical Association.* 1951; 147:1629-1635.

27. Chandler, G. Deleterious effect of intra-articular hydrocortisone. *Lancet.* 1958; 2:661.

28. Chunekamrai, S. Changes in articular cartilage after intra-articular injections of methylprednisolone acetate in horses. *American Journal of Veterinary Research.* 1989; 50:1733-1741.

29. Rusanen, M. Scanning electron microscopial study of the effects of crystalloid and water-soluble glucocorticoids on articular cartilage. *Scand J Rheumatology.* 1986; 15: 47-51.

CHAPTER 2

The Verdict: Nope to Scope!

"...I will follow that method of treatment which, according to my ability and judgement, I consider for the benefit of my patients, and abstain from whatever is deleterious and mischievous..."
–Hippocratic Oath

Even high-powered professional teams have orthopedic surgeons as their team physicians, whose healing tools primarily consist of **RICE**, NSAIDs, cortisone shots, the arthroscope, and the scalpel. Which one of these actually heals or repairs the injury? The answer is none of them. None of these treatments repairs the injury. What they actually do is weaken or "damage" the athlete and decrease the chances of healing. It is a sad fact that after the team physician has gone through the arsenal of **RICE**, anti-inflammatories, and cortisone shots, the infamous "scope recommendation" will soon follow for the non-healing athletic injury. (A sad commentary of the average sports medicine physician is seen in ***Figure 2-1***.) The problem is that athletes have no idea what is involved with arthroscopy. Guess what orthopedists call it? Arthroscopic **surgery**. Arthroscopy is surgery. If an athlete wants surgery, arthroscopy is a good place to start. This is a warning: there is no such thing as a "take a look" arthroscopy. Arthroscopy with big scopes almost **always involves shaving, cutting, and sewing**. There is generally very little sewing, and a lot of bzzz, bzzz, bzzz. It isn't your stubble falling off of a barber's razor either. It is the meniscus, cartilage, and ligaments that are getting buzzed. The myth that athletes have been fed is that a scope can find out the problem and solve it. Nothing could be farther from the truth for the average sports injury. All the arthroscope can do is look at the tissue. That is it. A physician or allied health care provider, and preferably one familiar with ligaments, tendons, and Prolotherapy, can tell you what is causing the pain.[1] That is it. X-rays, MRIs, or arthroscopies cannot show the actual problem. All they can do is show a picture that is not necessarily the cause of the problem.

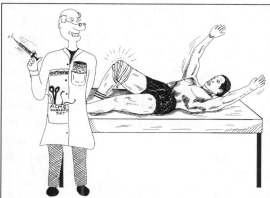

Figure 2-1: The Injured Athlete's Nightmare
The "Tools" an orthopedic surgeon uses to "fix" athletic injuries, such as NSAIDs, cortisone, and the arthroscope, actually ***cause*** more damage.

ARTHROSCOPY:
THE QUICKEST ROUTE TO AN ATHLETIC INJURY

The easiest and most overt way athletes are injured is not from a cheap shot from an opponent, but by one of their supposed allies, the arthroscope. This subtle stoic instrument is slipped into the knees, ankles, and shoulders of athletes while they are asleep. The subtle intruder, so innocent, so shiny, unknown to the athlete, has razor-sharp teeth that slice through tissue easier than the slick blade of a butcher. The arthroscope is capable of producing more irreversible damage than the most vicious opponent produces. The damage is, however, often masked by the incredible feeling of vitality following the procedure. The athlete's euphoria, because someone has finally fixed the problem is followed by a tenacious rehabilitation course, as the athlete is eager to get back to the field. The problem is that the scope did nothing but make the athlete's knee, shoulder, ankle, or whatever joint **weaker**. The weakness is masked by the massive amount of exercise that the athlete does after the procedure. The athlete experiences continued pain, but the orthopedist insists that more exercise is needed. The athletes often return to their sports, perhaps with less pain than before the scope, but report that their joints "just never felt the same" after the surgery. There is a sense that something is not quite right, but they cannot put a finger on it. This is a sure sign that weakness is the cause of that "just not quite right" feeling. The knee is now weaker. The shoulder is now weaker. The ankle is now weaker. This is why the athlete does not feel quite right.

WHAT IS ARTHROSCOPY?

The word arthroscopy comes from the prefix arth-, which means joint, and scope, which means scope. Arthroscopy involves inserting a scope into a joint to look at it. The guise under which arthroscopy flourishes is that it is supposed to help with diagnosis of an athlete's problem and allows the orthopedist the ability to fix the problem immediately. This is reiterated in one of the main sports medicine textbooks available today, in the following, "The most important factor in the treatment of any athletic injury is the ability of the physician to make a quick, accurate diagnosis. The appropriate treatment plan, correct prognosis, and potential for return to activity by the patient all depend on the accuracy of the initial diagnosis. The availability of the arthroscope has much improved our diagnostic skills. Other sophisticated diagnostic modalities have also evolved, and magnetic resonance imaging (MRI), in particular, has in many instances proven better for diagnosing injuries, because it is non-invasive and provides a complete picture of interstitial lesions as well as lesions of bone, cartilage, and ligament. Although the arthroscope remains valuable as a diagnostic tool, its therapeutic modality for joint disorders is the single most important factor in the advancement of care of athletic injuries.[2]

With teaching like this, is it any wonder that an arthroscope is an orthopedist's best friend? Their logic for making a proper diagnosis with the arthroscope and the MRI is flawed. What about the orthopedist? The orthopedist's arthroscope is considered the number one advancement in sports medicine in the past 20 years. What a sad statement for the sports medicine field. A more proper statement is "...for the sports **surgery** field." Orthopedists are called team physicians, but should more appropriately be called team **surgeons**. A non-surgically oriented physician should fill the role as the true team physician. The arthroscopy is the greatest advance in the last 20 years in the surgical approach to the athletic injuries. The most important factor for the advancement of the non-surgical care of athletic injuries is Prolotherapy.

It is important to know exactly what is involved in receiving arthroscopy. It is a surgical procedure. The majority of arthroscopic surgeries in the United States are currently performed with either spinal block or general anesthesia.[2] This means that the person is totally anesthetized (knocked out) or paralyzed from the waist down (spinal block). These procedures obviously carry their own risks.

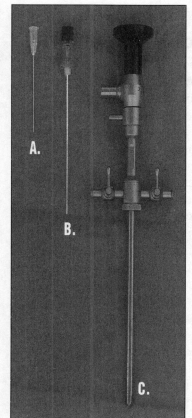

Figure 2-2: Comparison of the Prolotherapy Needle (A.) versus Spinal Needle (B.) versus Arthroscope (C.)
—Which would you rather have pierce your knee?

The following instruments are normally needed to perform arthroscopic procedures:

1. 4.0-mm diameter arthroscope with a 30-degree viewing lens
2. 4.0-mm diameter arthroscope with a 70-degree viewing lens
3. Video camera
4. Recorder
5. Pump
6. Motorized shavers or bur (a rotary cutting instrument)
7. Probe
8. Assorted hand instruments (e.g., grasper, clamps, curette).[2]

At any one time during arthroscopy of the knee, four instruments could be stuck into an athlete's knee—including scopes, probes, shavers, pumps, and various other instruments of local destruction. *(See Figure 2-2.)* The question to ask is how can so many instruments be stuck into such a small space? This is a great question. The knee joint normally contains only a small amount of fluid, approximately five millimeters. During a scope, one of the ports (place for a probe) is for the pump. This device pumps saline water into the knee. Depending on the knee, up to 120 milliliters of fluid may be pumped into the knee under force. The question to ask is would not ballooning up the knee to this degree cause the ligaments, meniscus, cartilage, and joints to become stretched, inflamed, and injured? Could it be possible that this forceful pumping of fluid in-and-of-itself might cause the tears, rough edges, and inflammation that are so often reported on arthroscopy reports? What about the presence of all of these probes, shavers, and other instruments in such a small area? The tissue of the knee might be damaged, as water is pumped under pressure and inserted into the knee. What stops the instruments from moving around? Imagine an athlete's knee 10 to 20 times the normal size. That is what the knee looks like during arthroscopy. *(See Figure 2-3.)* Are you having any doubts about arthroscopy yet? You should!

Another interesting question is, perhaps, what are the benefits of arthroscopy? What is meant by this question is, does arthroscopy produce immediate pain relief, often experienced after the surgery, or are these results from the joint being flushed? The question has already been asked and answered.

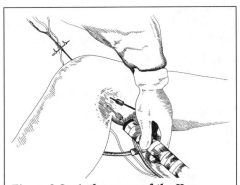

Figure 2-3: Arthroscopy of the Knee
The procedure involves "blowing up" the knee 10 to 20 times its normal size, and then generally shearing, removing, and cutting tissue. Does this sound like it's in the best interest of the athlete?

ARTHROSCOPY VERSUS JOINT LAVAGE: A COMPARISON STUDY

Rowland Chang, M.D., and associates at Northwestern University in Chicago, conducted a study to compare arthroscopic surgery to joint lavage in treating people with chronic knee pain. The patients had persistent knee pain for longer than three months and, despite conservative medical and rehabilitation management, remained work-restricted and unable to perform athletic or self-care activities to an extent acceptable to the patient. The patients were divided into two groups: one group received a joint lavage and the other group received arthroscopy. The joint lavage involved inserting a needle into the knee and flushing the joint with about 1,000 milliliters of fluid. The patients were seen at three months post-procedure and again at 12 months. At three months, 50 percent of the arthroscopy group exhibited improvement and 42 percent experienced improvement in the joint lavage group.

However, at 12 months, 44 percent of the arthroscopy group and 58 percent of the joint lavage group exhibited improvement. The authors concluded, "At three months of follow-up, there were no significant between-group differences in pain, self-reported and observed functional status, and patient and "blinded" physician global assessments. After one year, 44 percent of the subjects who underwent arthroscopy reported improvement and 58 percent of subjects who underwent joint lavage improved."[3] The authors further concluded,

"The widespread use of MRI or office arthroscopy cannot be recommended without data indicating that these procedures can accurately determine arthroscopically detectable meniscal lesions and that arthroscopic surgery is more effective than lavage in this particular subset of patients."[3]

Perhaps the most important fact is that when this study was done in 1987 the average charge for arthroscopy at a non-teaching, not-for-profit community hospital was $5,000.00. The lavage, which was performed in the physician's office, cost $660. The authors noted that the differential cost for the arthroscopy procedure relative to lavage was therefore $3840. This also excluded time lost from work because of the arthroscopy and all of the ancillary charges along with it, in addition to the costs of rehabilitation after the surgery was completed.[3]

There are many important points to this study. Arthroscopy is effective at eliminating the pain in about 50 percent of the people, yet the same effect is obtained by going to the physician's office and flushing the knee. In addition, you save about $4,000 and can go right back to work. This study also makes you wonder if the initial benefit of arthroscopy is not just due to the joint flushing. If it were our knee and we had the choice between the two procedures, we would certainly go for the joint flushing. It is a whole lot less invasive and less expensive. See *Figure 2-4* comparing the two.

It turns out that the use of saline irrigation of the knee is over 50 years old. In 1949, M. Watanabe, M.D., showed that articular pumping, or lavaging of the knee, could eliminate knee pain.[4] It is truly unfortunate for the athletes that simple, effective techniques like joint flushing and Prolotherapy are not more utilized, especially when they have been shown to work. Another interesting fact about joint flushing is that it has been shown to be more effective than NSAIDs for treatment of arthritis of the knee. In one study involving seven medical centers and eight physicians' offices, knee irrigation was shown to be statistically **more effective** than traditional medical management for knee arthritis in improving pain, stiffness, and function of people with arthritis of the knee.[5] Other researchers have also shown the same effects with knee lavage.[6]

ARTHROSCOPY VERSUS JOINT LAVAGE

	ARTHROSCOPIC SURGERY	JOINT LAVAGE
TIME	HOURS	MINUTES
INSTRUMENTS USED	PROBES	NEEDLES
NUMBER OF PROBES/NEEDLES TO BE STUCK INTO KNEE	FOUR	TWO
ANESTHESIA	SPINAL/GENERAL	LOCAL
REHABILITATION	EXTENSIVE	MINIMAL
COST	$5,000 +	LESS THAN $1,000
RESPONSE	50%	50%

Figure 2-4: *Arthroscopy versus Joint Lavage*
The above information makes you wonder if perhaps the "benefits" from arthroscopy are simply due to the joint being flushed or lavaged. So the question is—why not just flush the joint?

EARLY ARTHROSCOPIC COMPLICATIONS

As seen in *Figures 2-2 and 2-3*, arthroscopy involves the prodding of four-millimeter arthroscopes throughout the knee. Three probes are generally used, producing three scars after arthroscopy. The procedure itself is not without complications. In a large multi-center study, the types of complications associated with arthroscopy were tabulated.[7] These are shown in *Figure 2-5*.

The most common complication is bleeding into the joint after the arthroscopy. This is expected because the knee joint is pumped with 100 milliliters of fluid and then three large probes are inserted. Infection accounted for 12.1 percent of the complications and blood clots (thromboembolic disease) accounted for 6.9 percent.

TYPES OF COMPLICATIONS

COMPLICATION	PERCENTAGE	NUMBER
Hemarthrosis/Hematoma	60.1	104
Infection	12.1	21
Thromboembolic disease	6.9	12
Anesthetic	6.4	11
Instrument failure	2.9	5
Reflex sympathetic dystrophy	2.3	4
Ligament injury	1.2	2
Fracture	0.6	1
Neurologic injury	0.6	1
Miscellaneous	6.9	12
Vascular injury	0.0	0
Total	**100.0**	**173**

Figure 2-5: Complications Tabulated In One Arthroscopic Study
Hemarthrosis or bleeding into the joint, along with infections, are the most common complications from arthroscopic surgery.

It should be noted that specific kinds of arthroscopic procedures have their own kinds of complications. For instance, in ACL reconstruction (ligament reconstruction of the knee) all of the following types of complications have been reported: hemarthrosis, hematoma (blood clot), sepsis, skin necrosis, arthrofibrosis (excessive scar tissue), deep venous thrombosis (vein blood clot), recurrent effusion (fluid keeps filling in the knee), sensory nerve injury, reflex sympathetic dystrophy (formation of severe chronic knee pain), tourniquet paralysis, tissue irritation over a metallic device, and compartmental syndrome.[8] The most common complication in ACL reconstruction, however, is arthrofibrosis, resulting in loss of flexion, extension, or both. This means that, after the arthroscopy, the person cannot move the knee normally. It is fibrosed, or scarred down, so normal movement is not possible. The incidence of this has been shown to be as high as 3.7 percent.[8, 9] ACL reconstruction complications also occur due to use of the synthetic or natural grafts. Some people react to both the synthetic and natural grafts and reject them.

Arthroscopic meniscal repair is no cakewalk either, with a 2.4 percent complication rate. One study reported 30 saphenous nerve injuries, six peroneal nerve injuries, 22 infections, three vascular injuries (injury to blood vessels), and four cases of thrombophlebitis (irritation or infection of blood vessels).[10]

Lateral retinacular release, a common arthroscopic procedure for chondromalacia patella (cartilage deterioration beneath the kneecap) is the grandaddy of complication-ridden procedures. This is a very common procedure given to athletes because of so-called "bad kneecap tracking" onto the femur. Some studies report up to a 9.2 percent complication rate.[8, 11] The surgery sometimes makes the kneecap so unstable that it starts to move medially (toward the center) because too much of the soft tissue was cut.

Shoulder arthroscopy is also fraught with complications. Complications have included nerve injury, rotator cuff tears, as well as the usual hemarthrosis and infections.[8, 12]

The take home point, here, is that when several large probes are inserted into the knee, shoulder, ankle, elbow, or some other joint, bad things can happen. Infections, bleeding, nerve injury, blood vessel damage, and even damage to the structures in the injured joint itself may occur. The athlete has the choice: scope using several large probes or Prolotherapy or joint lavage using needles. It may be wise to review the pictures in the center of the book to compare the techniques. The choice is yours. The answer seems very obvious, but for some, the pressure to scope is just too much. Remember what Nancy Reagan said, "Just say no!"

DOES ARTHROSCOPY CURE ANYTHING?

The main concerns for the injured person should be to find medical procedures or drugs that cure the problem. It was evident from the preceding chapters that NSAIDs and cortisone shots do not cure anything and have detrimental effects on the body. They have harmful effects because they stop normal healing by decreasing inflammation. What do you think will happen when you remove tissue from a knee even if it is torn? There can be only one answer and the answer is not good, especially for the athlete.

MENISCAL INJURY

The menisci consist of semilunar fibrocartilage, partly filling the space between the femoral and tibial bones. Four principal functions are ascribed to the menisci: *(See Figure 2-6a and 6b.)*

1. To spread a thin film of synovial fluid which provides nutrition to the articular cartilage
2. To act as shock absorbers
3. To increase the stability of the knee joint
4. To aid in the complex rotatory mechanics of the knee joint[13]

Meniscus injuries occur in most sports, but most commonly occur in contact sports. They often occur in combination with ligament injuries, particularly when the medial meniscus is involved. This is partly because the medial meniscus is attached to the medial collateral ligament and partly because tackles are often directed towards the lateral side of the knee, causing external rotation of the tibia. *(See Figure 2-7.)* Injury to the medial meniscus is about five times more common than injury to the lateral meniscus.[14]

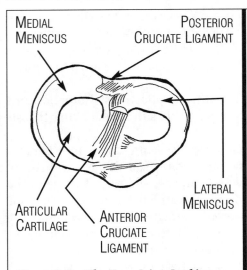

MEDIAL MENISCUS

POSTERIOR CRUCIATE LIGAMENT

LATERAL MENISCUS

ARTICULAR CARTILAGE

ANTERIOR CRUCIATE LIGAMENT

Figure 2-6a: The Knee Joint, Looking from the Top
Anatomy inside the knee shows the posterior cruciate ligament, anterior cruciate ligament, medial meniscus, and lateral meniscus.

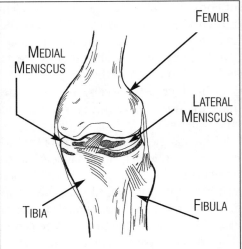

FEMUR

MEDIAL MENISCUS

LATERAL MENISCUS

FIBULA

TIBIA

Figure 2-6b: Anatomy of the Knee, Looking from Behind
The menisci (lateral and medial) cushion the joint between the tibia and femur bones.

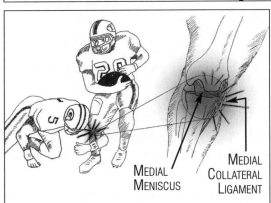

MEDIAL MENISCUS

MEDIAL COLLATERAL LIGAMENT

Figure 2-7: Injury to the Medial Meniscus During Contact Sports
A hit on the the knee causing a medial meniscus and medial collateral ligament injury. If the hit is severe enough, the anterior cruciate ligament will also be torn.

By knowing the function of the meniscus, it is possible to predict what will happen when meniscal tissue is shaved or removed. Since it provides some of the nutrition to the articular cartilage, its removal will aid in the demise of the cartilage. If the cartilage is damaged, then the pressures on the bone will be too great and arthritis will soon follow. This is not the only reason why articular cartilage damage is sure to follow after meniscectomy. The removal of the menisci allows too much pressure to be put on the articular cartilage, thus lessening the shock absorption. This is why cartilage damage and proliferative arthritis must be the end result of meniscal removal. No other option is available. If the surgeon removes the meniscus, arthritis is the end result. If that were not enough, the menisci aid in the stability of the knee. If they are removed, the knee is left with too much motion and becomes unstable. This

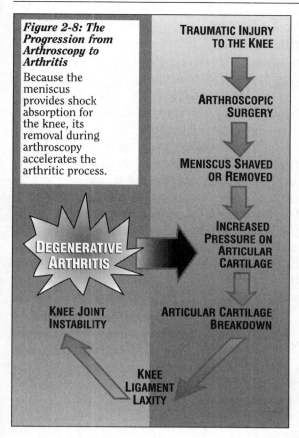

Figure 2-8: The Progression from Arthroscopy to Arthritis

Because the meniscus provides shock absorption for the knee, its removal during arthroscopy accelerates the arthritic process.

TRAUMATIC INJURY TO THE KNEE

ARTHROSCOPIC SURGERY

MENISCUS SHAVED OR REMOVED

INCREASED PRESSURE ON ARTICULAR CARTILAGE

DEGENERATIVE ARTHRITIS

KNEE JOINT INSTABILITY

ARTICULAR CARTILAGE BREAKDOWN

KNEE LIGAMENT LAXITY

also increases the likelihood of articular cartilage damage and subsequent arthritis. *(See Figure 2-8.)*

Arthroscopic shaving and removal of the meniscus would therefore be expected to result in the progression of arthritis in the knee. Prolotherapy, on the other hand, would be expected to heal the meniscus, since Prolotherapy stimulates the body to repair the injured tissue. Prolotherapy given to the injured menisci stimulates fibroblastic growth of new stronger meniscal tissue, thereby repairing the area. This makes a lot more sense than its removal.

STUDY SHOWS INCREASED CONTACT STRESS PRESSURE AFTER MENISCECTOMY

There have been numerous studies showing that the contact stress pressure on the articular cartilage significantly increases after meniscal removal.[15, 16] One such study showed that after partial meniscectomy, the contact stress pressures increased by 110 percent and after total meniscectomy they increased 200 percent. Their conclusion was expected. "The contact stresses increased in proportion to the amount of meniscus removed.[17] Other studies have shown even greater increases in pressure, causing from a 450 to 600 percent (six times) increase in pressure on the tibia bone and articular cartilage when the meniscus is removed.[18, 19]

Menisci are normally shaved or removed because they are believed to repair so poorly. Menisci, like many of the soft tissues treated with Prolotherapy, have poor blood supply. This is one of the reasons they heal poorly. The best treatment option is to increase the circulation to the damaged menisci. Athletes with meniscal injuries are generally given RICE treatment, which dramatically further decreases circulation to the damaged menisci. The MEAT protocol and Prolotherapy, on the other hand, improves blood circulation to the damaged area and stimulates repair.

STUDIES SHOW MENISCAL SURGERY ACTUALLY *INCREASES* INJURY

Repairing a meniscal tear with arthroscopy makes conceptual sense, however, this just does not occur often enough to warrant the procedure. In an animal study, only 38 percent of the meniscal repairs actually healed.[20] To add insult to injury, another study showed that meniscal repair can actually cause a further spreading of the injury to the non-injured meniscal tissue. The authors noted, "It appears that in radial repairs, progressive spreading at the repair site altered normal meniscal geometry and structure, adversely influencing mechanical function."[21] In common language, attempting to repair the area with arthroscopy makes the normal meniscal tissue weaker and further worsens the injury. The authors went on to say, "Meniscal tissue from repaired radial lesions was significantly lower than controls in yield stress, maximum stress, and elastic modulus. The repaired radial meniscal lesions demonstrated abnormal force transmission and energy dissipation behavior qualitatively similar to a complete meniscectomy."[21] This is unbelievable! Repairing a meniscal tear makes the meniscal tissue so weak that it is like having no menisci at all. What a scary thought!

INCOMPLETE HEALING AND FURTHER DETERIORATION RESULT AFTER MENISCAL REPAIR SURGERY

In one large study, where 82 percent of the meniscal injuries were sustained from sporting events, a full 75 percent of the meniscal repairs did not completely heal.[22] The follow-up arthroscopic examinations were done at a mean of 18 months and clinical examinations at 42 months. This is one and a half and three and a half years later, folks. These are not impressive statistics to encourage athletes to undergo meniscal repairs. In this study, in only 18 months, 20 percent of the patients had articular cartilage damage on the tibia and femur that was not present on the initial arthroscopy, but was seen in follow-up arthroscopy. A full 40 percent had deterioration of the articular cartilage under the knee cap.[22] This deterioration occurred over only 18 months! Yet the authors of the paper state that 80 percent of the patients were asymptomatic. But 20 percent of the patients needed further arthroscopic surgery! You see the difference between pain-free and healed? Athletes are being coerced into these procedures that do not repair or heal the injured the tissue. Eighty percent were pain-free **while** their cartilage was rapidly deteriorating. What is being done to stop this arthritic process? Unless the orthopedist plans to refer the athlete for Prolotherapy, nothing is being done.

MENISCECTOMY CAUSES ARTHRITIS

Repairing meniscal tears does not work; neither does grafting tissue over the tear. In one study on sheep knees, one group received a total meniscectomy, two groups received different grafts, and the control group received no surgery.

Guess which group did better? You guessed it! The virgin knee group that was never probed by a scope fared the best. On follow-up x-ray after only 21 months, the control knees had no arthritis, but the meniscectomized knees had significant arthritis in all the compartments of the knee, as well as the grafted knees. The authors concluded, "Knees undergoing each of the three procedures in our study showed significant degenerative changes when compared with the non-operated control knees. This would suggest that **surgical intrusion into the knee predisposes it to osteoarthritic changes."**[23] What a shock!

PARTIAL MENISCECTOMY: MORE ARTHRITIC CHANGES RESULT

Luis Bolano, M.D., and associates at the Oklahoma Center for Athletes and the University of Oklahoma wanted to determine the long-term results of arthroscopic partial meniscectomy. They noted that the short-term results of arthroscopic partial meniscectomy had been excellent-to-good in 80 to 95 percent of patients in the already published studies.[24] What they found surprised them. The patients, many of whom were athletes, were functioning fairly well. Eighty percent experienced satisfactory results, 66 percent maintained their activity levels, but 26 percent decreased their activity levels after the surgery. Despite the apparent success of the surgery, almost all of the patients showed arthritic changes on x-ray. Forty-one percent had advanced arthritis. The authors noted, "The amount of meniscus removed and the type of tear had a significant effect on the radiographic result."[24]

The problem with arthroscopic surgery is that it does not induce the healing of the menisci. The athlete feels better for a while, but the injured tissue remains injured. This causes the arthritic process to start immediately. If left unchecked, the athlete's abilities will decline, symptomatology will increase, and more arthroscopic or orthopedic surgeries will follow. If the athletes want this, then by all means, continue to be scoped. If they want to avoid arthritis, they must see a Prolotherapist and receive Prolotherapy to stimulate the body to heal the menisci and other injured tissue.

THE OUTLOOK IS NOT GOOD FOR POST-SURGICAL ATHLETES

What is the outlook down the road, 12 to 15 years, for people who have had arthroscopic partial meniscectomies? Not good. In a study of 21 patients who had partial meniscectomy, six needed further meniscal surgery and seven required additional knee surgery. Over 50 percent of the meniscectomized knees needed knee surgery by 12 to 15 years down the road. Eighteen of the 21 patients who underwent meniscectomy had arthritis in the knee. The three with no arthritis were, likely, very inactive people. About 50 percent of the knees, however, had advanced arthritis compared to the non-operated knees. This statement by the authors should be of significance to the athletes, "The activity level of the patients in both groups changed...indicating a downward change from active individual sports, such as tennis, squash, or downhill skiing, to less strenuous physical fitness activities such as cycling, hiking, or cross-country skiing."[25]

Other studies have confirmed similar findings. If no cartilage deterioration occurred before meniscus removal, deterioration will occur after the surgery.[26] Long-term effects of meniscus removal lead to increased contact stresses and subsequent articular cartilage degeneration.[27-30]

It is time for athletes to take a stand, even under intense pressure, and say, "The verdict is in: say nope to scope!" Your long-term health may be dramatically altered once the scope enters your knee. At least in meniscal injuries, arthroscopies do not cure anything.

ANTERIOR CRUCIATE LIGAMENT INJURIES

Some of the most horrible words a competitive athlete could hear are, "You have an anterior cruciate ligament tear." All of the treatment options for this condition stink. In the best case scenario, athletes are told that a tendon can replace the ligament and the rehabilitation of this new structure takes a full year. Maybe the athlete will be able to compete again at a later date. In an international sports medicine journal, they put it this way, "The competitive elite athlete who sustains an anterior cruciate ligament (ACL) rupture has few options for treatment. If they wish to continue to compete at the pre-injury level, then the only viable option is to undergo an ACL reconstruction. Otherwise, the athlete with an ACL deficient knee is at substantial risk of sustaining subsequent degenerative changes in the knee at a young age.[31]

Ligament injuries in the knee should be treated as potentially serious since they provide for the stability of the knee. They are as common as meniscus injuries and mainly affect athletes involved in contact sports such as football, ice hockey, team handball, basketball, rugby, and also Alpine skiing.[14] Ligament injuries in the knee occur mainly as the result of collisions with opponents during contact sports, but they also occur without body contact, with twisting and other movements that exceed the normal range of motion. The various ligaments of the knee joints cooperate in order to maintain the stability of the joint. The stronger the stresses put on the joint, the greater the degree to which the ligaments are engaged. A ligament combination is often injured because of this fact. Perhaps the most common injury involves the triad of ligaments: the medial meniscus (ligament), medial collateral (ligament), and anterior cruciate (ligament). This occurs because the knee is generally hit from the lateral (outside) side, which forces the knee to buckle inward, injuring those three ligaments. *(Refer back to Figure 2-7.)*

ACL TEARS: SOME OF THE WORST INJURIES IMAGINABLE

ACL (anterior cruciate ligament) tears are some of the most common sports injuries. A typical scenario is this: An athlete involved in an agility sport decelerates and pivots on a planted foot especially when trying to pivot around an opponent, feels a pop in the knee, falls, and is unable to continue play. *(See*

Figure 2-9.) Within an hour, the knee swells. X-rays in the emergency room that night are read as negative. The athlete is prescribed **RICE** treatments and an anti-inflammatory medication. After several weeks, the swelling resolves, the pain subsides, and the athlete returns to play. The athlete thinks the doctors and therapists are incredible for the great treatment received. A short time later, the athlete reinjures the knee. The athlete again thinks that he must not be training enough. In reality, the second injury occurred because the original injury never healed. Remember pain relief is not the goal, a healed injury is the goal.

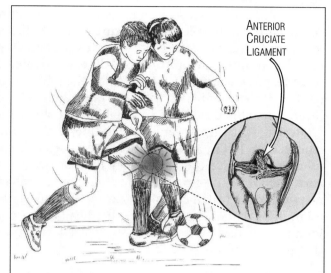

ANTERIOR CRUCIATE LIGAMENT

Figure 2-9: *Mechanism of Anterior Cruciate Ligament Injury in Agility Sports*
When trying to pivot around an opponent, an athlete decelerates and pivots on on a planted foot, causing the ACL injury.

ACL TEARS: TO TREAT OR NOT TO TREAT— THE CHOICES ARE NOT GOOD

ACL tears are so significant because, if left untreated, they have terrible consequences and, if treated, there are bad consequences. It is crucial for the athlete to make the correct choice. Unfortunately the choices are usually between which is the lesser of two evils. If the athlete knows about Prolotherapy, which is the only treatment for ACL tears that actually helps the body repair the injured area, a good choice will be made.

An untreated ACL deficient knee is unstable and arthritis eventually forms. One study following people with ACL tears that were treated non-operatively showed that 86 percent felt the knee giving way at four-years' follow-up. A full return to unlimited athletic activities was possible for only 14 percent.[32] In another study with about 10 years follow-up, 78 percent of the knees treated without surgery showed osteoarthritis.[33] Other studies have confirmed that, besides giving way, ACL deficient knees are plagued by swelling and stiffness long term.[34] The most significant finding for most of the studies is that ACL deficient athletes seldom come back to playing their athletics at the same level. In one study, 72 percent of the athletes had problems with walking, running, turning, cutting, jumping, or climbing stairs 18 months after the injury.[34]

The sad part about ACL injuries is that the injured athlete is usually very young with a full career in the future. Most studies involve athletes who want to return to their athletic events, but few seldom do with this type of injury. In one long-term follow-up study of ACL tears, treated conservatively over a four to 10 year follow-up, only 20 percent of the athletes returned to their pre-injury level of athletic activities without restrictions. The rest had arthritis. Eighty-seven percent had evidence of instability on physical examination.[35]

Realize that the conservative treatments the athletes received in the above studies were **RICE**, anti-inflammatories, cortisone shots, physical therapy, and other conservative therapies. They did not receive that treatment that could **cure** them, which is Prolotherapy. Prolotherapy can cure a partial ACL tear, but not a complete tear. A complete tear requires surgery. Prolotherapy is still helpful in this situation, because the other ligaments around the knee, as well as the joint capsule itself, were at least stretched during the forceful event to the knee that totally disrupted the ACL.

WHAT ABOUT ACL SURGERY?

The standard of care for ACL tears today is surgery. There are various surgical techniques employed in the ACL reconstruction: repair through the patellar defect, arthroscopically-assisted techniques, and the mini-arthrotomy technique. According to one well-known source, "...these techniques all give both excellent and reproducible results."[31] The problem is that the orthopedic surgeons' views on excellent results is different than the athletes' views. The athlete is thinking "I'm going to be back to my sport as good as new as soon as the surgery is over." The orthopedist is thinking, "This athlete doesn't have a chance to be back on that ball field, but the surgery will help stabilize the knee." Poor communication is at the crux of this. The final goals and desired outcomes are never discussed.

ACL reconstruction surgery involves surgically placing a prosthesis or a tendon in the place of the injured ligament. The question to ask is, "Will this surgery allow me to return to athletics?" To answer this question athletes were followed for an average of nine years at the Sports Medicine Facility of Health Sciences at Linkoping University, in Sweden, by Dr. W. Maletius and associates. ACL replacement was performed with Dacron prostheses. In the nine year period, 65 percent of the patients required another arthroscopy. Forty percent had meniscal problems that were treated arthroscopically. At the nine year follow-up only 48 percent of the patients had intact menisci. Forty-four percent of the prostheses had ruptured during the follow-up period. Eighty-three percent of the patients had significant arthritic changes on x-ray in the operated knee. The authors concluded, "Based on the functional results of the patients with a ligament in place after nine years, only 14 percent of the original group had acceptable stability and knee function."[36] Some authors have claimed that prosthetic ACL substitution is an "iatrogenic model" of degenerative arthritis in the human knee.[37]

Surgical technique has improved and perhaps the gold standard for ACL reconstruction today is to use the patellar tendon to replace the injured ACL. The surgeon takes some of the patellar tendon and screws it into the femur and tibia bones to simulate an anterior cruciate ligament. The long-term results are better than Dacron prosthesis, but are still not that great. In one five year study of arthroscopic anterior cruciate ligament reconstruction with patellar tendon graft showed that 5 percent of the patients ruptured their grafts. Of the remaining patients, about 50 percent had symptoms in their knees. Of significance to athletes was that 53 percent of them could perform at the same or a better level at five years post surgery. This means that 47 percent were performing at a lower level of activity.[38] The authors interestingly discussed, "In the literature, there has been a lack of documentation that reconstructing an ACL-deficient knee prevents arthritic changes."[38] In another study following the patients for seven years, a slightly longer period of time, only 46 percent of the athletes could perform at the same level as their pre-injury status. In this study 26 percent needed another operative procedure after the ACL reconstruction.[39]

Substituting the real ACL for an artificial one will never be ideal. The tendon grafts have been found to be three to four times stiffer than normal ACLs and artificial graft particles have been shown to cause proliferative arthritis when injected into knees.[40, 41] The athlete's best option is always to first try stimulating the ACL to repair itself. Case reports of complete tears healing without any treatment have been reported in the literature.[42] A much better approach is to receive Prolotherapy for ACL tears. Prolotherapy can be done exactly where the ACL attaches onto the tibia and femur, thereby stimulating the ligament on both ends to proliferate and strengthen. It is only then, by the strengthening of the ACL, will the athlete truly be healed.

For the athlete who puts hope in ACL reconstruction surgery, the road will be a long one. Even if the surgery is successful, a full year of intense rehabilitation is generally needed. Patellar tendon autographs do not achieve full strength evidently until nine months after surgery.[43] An athlete should also realize that a functional knee brace must be worn for 15 to 18 months post-operatively, according to most orthopedists.[44] If the graft is so strong, why would an athlete have to wear a brace? The answer is that the grafts are not that strong. Other researchers have noticed that a high percentage of knees become lax (weak) more than two years postoperatively.[45] The best option for the athlete is to try Prolotherapy to the ACL. Even Prolotherapists are often amazed at how quickly the athlete rockets back once the proliferation of the ligament takes hold.

ARTHROSCOPY FOR ARTHRITIS IS CALLED SHAM

I changed the title somewhat. It actually read, "A Knee Surgery for Arthritis is Called Sham." This was the title of one of the lead articles in the *New York Times,* July 11, 2002 by Gina Kolata.[48] Gina wrote:

A popular operation for arthritis of the knee worked no better than a sham procedure in which patients were sedated while surgeons pretended to operate, researchers are reporting today.

The operation—arthroscopic surgery for the pain and stiffness caused by osteoarthritis— is done on at least 225,000 middle-age and older Americans each year at a cost of more than a billion dollars to Medicare, the Department of Veterans Affairs and private insurers.

In the study, to be published today in The New England Journal of Medicine, investigators at the Houston Veterans Affairs Medical Center and Baylor College of Medicine report that while patients often said they felt better after surgery, their improvement was just wishful thinking. Tests of knee functions revealed that the operation had not helped, and those who got the placebo surgery reported feeling just as good as those who had had the real operation.

"Here we are doing all this surgery on people and it's all a sham," said Dr. Baruch Brody, an ethicist at Baylor who helped design the study.

In the actual summary from The New England Journal of Medicine article the authors said "In this controlled trial involving patients with osteoarthritis of the knee, the outcomes after arthroscopic lavage or arthroscopic debridement were not better than after a placebo procedure."

In other words, arthroscopic surgery for arthritis doesn't work. Two days after the above report the Arthroscopy Association of North America wrote,

When arthritis is a component of the problem in the knee, it is well recognized that arthroscopic techniques have limitations. When it is obvious by x-rays and physical examination that arthritis in the knee is advanced, arthroscopy should not be considered. If there is a narrowed joint space on x-ray, with no mechanical symptoms, arthroscopy offers the patient no chance of relief.[49]

Bravo! I concur. The next reasonable question is, why is this procedure still being done so frequently for arthritis then? Could it be greed-driven?

SUMMARY

Many people are scared to death when they become acutely injured. Before they know it, they are in an emergency room with strange people in white coats all staring at them. They are given the **RICE** treatment and anti-inflammatory medications. The orthopedic surgeon will then recommend an arthroscopy to "take a look" at the damage. The problem is that the scope is far more dangerous than the original traumatic injury. The arthroscopic procedure itself is fraught with potential complications, including hematoma and infection. The most dangerous effect, however, is the permanent weakness left in the joint when soft tissue structures, such as menisci are removed.

One of the most common arthroscopic procedures is partial meniscectomy, which has a high rate for development of long-term arthritis because of the high pressures generated on the tibial cartilage when the meniscus is removed. Anterior cruciate ligament (ACL) reconstruction is not much better, with a high percentage of athletes not returning to their pre-surgery level of athletics, even after a year of rehabilitation. Over 200,000 arthroscopies per year are done for degenerative joints. This procedure has been found to be a sham—and no better than a placebo. The reason for all of these suboptimal outcomes is because arthroscopy does not heal anything. Arthroscopy typically involves looking into the joint and shaving or removing tissue. This has nothing to do with repairing the damaged area. Even putting in artificial ligaments and tendon grafts, though helpful for some, is not truly repairing the area. Only Prolotherapy, by stimulating the actual proliferation (growth) of normal collagen tissue, will start the normal repair process of the injured ligaments and tendons. It is for this reason that many athletes are saying the verdict is in—"say nope to scope and yes to Prolotherapy." ∎

BIBLIOGRAPHY

1. Personal correspondence told to us on many occasions by Gustav A. Hemwall, M.D.
2. Baker, C. Arthroscopy in the treatment of knee disorders. In *The Hughston Clinic Sports Medicine Book*. Editor C. Baker, Baltimore, Maryland. Williams & Wilkins. 1995, pp. 538-542.
3. Chang, R. A randomized, controlled trial of arthroscopic surgery versus closed-needle joint lavage for patients with osteoarthritis of the knee. *Arthritis and Rheumatism*. 1993; 36:289-296.
4. Verweij, A. Arthroscopy: a method of diagnosing and evaluating degenerative processes in the knee joint. In: Verbrugge, G. Degenerative Joints: Test tubes, Tissues, Models, Man. Amsterdam: *Excerpta Medica*. 1982; 189-195.
5. Ike, R. Tidal irrigation versus conservative medical management in patients with osteoarthritis of the knee: a prospective randomized study. *The Journal of Rheumatology*. 1992; 19:772-779.
6. Jungmichel, D. (Joint washing—a treatment possibility in active arthritis) Gelenkwaschung—cinc behandlungsmoglichkeit bei aktivjerter arthrose. *Beitr Orthop Traumatol*. 1988; 35:512-517.
7. Small, N. Complications in arthroscopic surgery performed by experienced arthroscopists. *Arthroscopy*. 1989; 4:282.
8. Small, N. "Complications in arthroscopy." In *Complications in Orthopaedic Surgery*, Third Edition. Philadelphia, PA. J. B. Lippincott Company. 1994. pp. 1107-1118.
9. Malek, N. "Complications of ACL surgery." In *AAOS Summer Institute*, San Diego, California. 1988.
10. Crenshaw, A. *Campell's Operative Orthopedics*. St. Louis, MO: Mosby. 1992. pp. 1771-1773.
11. Hughston, J. Medial subluxation of the patella as a complication of lateral retinacular release. *American Journal of Sports Medicine*. 1988; 16:383.
12. Klein, A. Measurement of brachial plexus strain in arthroscopy of the shoulder. *Arthroscopy*. 1987; 3:45.
13. Brantigan, O. Mechanics of ligaments and menisci of knee joint. *Journal of Bone and Joint Surgery*. 1941; 23:44-46.
14. Peterson, L. *Sports Injuries*. Chicago, IL. *Year Book Medical Publishers*. 1983; pp. 296-299.
15. Ahmed, A. *In vitro* measurement of static pressure distribution in synovial joints. Part 1: Tibial surface of the knees. *Journal of Biomechanical Engineering*. 1983; 105:216-225.

16. Brown, T. *In vitro* contact stress distributions on the femoral condyles. *Journal of Orthopedic Research*. 1984; 2:190-199.

17. Baratz, M. Meniscal tears: The effect of meniscectomy and of repair on intra-articular contact areas and stress in the human knee. *American Journal of Sports Medicine*. 1986; 14:270-274.

18. Radin, E. Role of the menisci in the distribution of stress in the knee. *Clinical Orthopedics*. 1984; 185:290-294.

19. Seedom, B. Transmission of the load in the knee joint with special reference to the role of the menisci: Part 1. *Eng Med*. 1979; 8:220-228.

20. Cabaud, H. Medial meniscus repairs. *American Journal of Sports Medicine*. 1981; 9:129-134.

21. Newman, A. Mechanics of the healed meniscus in a canine model. *American Journal of Sports Medicine*. 1989; 17:164-175.

22. Rubman, M. Arthroscopic repair of meniscal tears that extend into the avascular zone. *American Journal of Sports Medicine*. 1998; 26:87-95.

23. Edwards, D. Radiographic changes in the knee after meniscal transplantation. *American Journal of Sports Medicine*. 1996; 24:222-229.

24. Bolano, L. Isolated arthroscopic partial meniscectomy. *American Journal of Sports Medicine*. 1993; 21:432-437.

25. Maletius, W. The effect of partial meniscectomy on the long-term prognosis of knees with localized, severe chondral damage. *American Journal of Sports Medicine*. 1996; 24:258-262.

26. Cox, J. The degenerative effects of partial and total resection of the medial meniscus in dogs' knees. *Clinical Orthopedics*. 1975; 109:178-183.

27. Allen, P. Later degenerative changes after medial meniscectomy. *Journal of Bone and Joint Surgery*. 1984; 66B:666-671.

28. Appel, H. Late results after meniscectomy in the knee joint. *Acta Orthop Scand* (Suppl). 1970, pg. 133.

29. Tapper, E. Late results after meniscectomy. *Journal of Bone and Joint Surgery*. 1969; 51A:517-526.

30. Veth, R. Clinical significance of knee joint changes after meniscectomy. *Clinical Orthopedics*. 1985; 198:56-60.

31. Shelbourne, K. Anterior cruciate ligament injury. *Sports Medicine*. 1994; 17:132-140.

32. Hawkins, R. Follow-up of the acute nonoperated isolated anterior cruciate ligament tear. *American Journal of Sports Medicine*. 1986; 4:205-210.

33. McDaniel, W. Untreated ruptures of the anterior cruciate ligament: A follow-up study. *Journal of Bone and Joint Surgery*. 1980; 62A:696-705.

34. Buckley, S. The natural history of conservatively treated partial anterior cruciate ligament tears. *American Journal of Sports Medicine*. 1989; 17:221-225.

35. Pattee, G. Four to ten year follow-up of unreconstructed anterior cruciate ligament tears. *American Journal of Sports Medicine*. 1989; 7:430-435.

36. Maletius, W. Long-term results of anterior cruciate ligament reconstruction with a Dacron prosthesis. *American Journal of Sports Medicine*. 1997; 25:288-293.

37. Klein, W. Synovitis and artificial ligaments. *Arthroscopy*. 1992; 8:116-124.

38. Otto, D. Five year results of single-incision arthroscopic anterior cruciate ligament reconstruction with patellar tendon autograft. *American Journal of Sports Medicine*. 1998; 26:181-188.

39. Bach, B. Arthroscopically assisted anterior cruciate ligament reconstruction using patellar tendon autograft. The *American Journal of Sports Medicine*. 1998; 26:20-29.

40. Noyes, F. Biochemical analysis of human ligament grafts used in knee-ligament repairs and reconstructions. The *Journal of Bone and Joint Surgery*. 1984; 66:344-352.

41. Olson, E. The biochemical and histological effects of artificial ligament wear particles: In vitro and in vivo studies. The *American Journal of Sports Medicine*. 1988; 16:558-602.

42. Kurosaka, M. Spontaneous healing of a tear of the anterior cruciate ligament. *The Journal of Bone and Joint Surgery*. 1998; 80A:1200-1203.

43. Clancy, W. Anterior and posterior cruciate ligament reconstruction in rhesus monkeys. *Journal of Bone and Joint Surgery*. 1981; 63A:1270-1284.

44. Wasilewski, S. Effect of surgical timing on return to sports activity after significant knee injuries. *Sports Medicine*. 1994; 18:156-161.

45. Barber-Westin, S. The effect of rehabilitation and return to activity on anterior-posterior knee displacements after anterior cruciate ligament reconstruction. *American Journal of Sports Medicine*. 1993; 21:264-270.

46. Burns, Thomas. Arthroscopic treatment of shoulder impingement in athletes. *American Journal of Sports Medicine*. 1992; 20:13-16.

47. Cordasco, F. Arthroscopic treatment of glenoid labral tears. *American Journal of Sports Medicine*. 1993; 21:425-430.

48. Moseley, J. A. Controlled Trial of Arthroscopic Surgery for Osteoarthritis of the Knee. *The New England Journal of Medicine*. 2002; 347: 81-88.

49. http://www.ana.org/membership/OAposition.html July 24, 2002 written by Burkhart, S.

CHAPTER 3

Inflammation: The Key to Healing the Injured Knee

During my fourth year of medical school, while on a dermatology rotation with four other medical students, I (Ross) had the opportunity to train under Gary Solomon, M.D., one of the most respected dermatologists in the country. Dr. Solomon told the class he was going to provide the secret to understanding human disease. If we knew the secret we would be leaps and bounds ahead of our colleagues and be masterful clinicians. I couldn't wait to hear it!

When that day finally arrived, Dr. Solomon explained that *inflammation* was the most important concept to understanding health and healing, especially in regard to the etiology and treatment of human ailments. Most clinicians do not understand inflammation, he said.

Inflammation?! Egads! Everyone knows about inflammation. At that time, I dismissed his comments and left disappointed. Years later when I learned about Prolotherapy, I realized Dr. Solomon had been right. Inflammation *is* the mechanism by which the body heals, regardless of the illness.

WHERE COMPLETE HEALING BEGINS

All human ailments, including ligament and tendon injury, involve inflammation. Inflammation is defined as the reaction of vascularized, living tissue to local injury.[1] The first stage of inflammation is the actual injury. Inflammation is the body's reaction to a local injury. Healing an injured area is dependent on the blood supplying inflammatory cells to repair the damaged tissue, which explains why vascularized, living tissue is crucial to the repair of any injured area. Vascularization refers to the blood supply to an area. Poor blood flow proportionately reduces healing. This is why the **R.I.C.E.** protocol should not be used but **M.E.A.T.** To assist the normal healing inflammatory reaction that occurs after a knee injury the person should do **m**ovement, **e**xercise, **a**nalgesics, and specific **t**reatments that promote healing such as heat, physiotherapy, ultrasound, and Prolotherapy. The analgesics include those that are not anti-healing such as digestive enzymes, bromelaine, or medications such as muscle relaxers or pain relieves like acetaminophen or Ultram. *(See Figure 3-1)*

Chronically weak ligaments and tendons are a result of inadequate repair following an injury and occur because of poor blood supply to the area where ligaments and tendons attach to the bone, the fibro-osseous junction.[2-4] *(See Figure 3-2.)* Due to the poor blood supply, the immune cells necessary to repair the affected area cannot reach the injury. Inadequate healing is the result. Nonsteroidal anti-inflammatory drugs (NSAIDs) and ice treatments decrease the blood flow even further, thus hampering the body's capability to heal the injured tissue.

RICE VERSUS MEAT

The RICE treatment leads to incomplete healing of soft tissue whereas MEAT encourages complete healing.

MODALITY	RESULT	MODALITY	RESULT
REST	Decreased joint nutrition	**M**OVEMENT	Increased joint nutrition
ICE	Decreased blood flow	**E**XERCISE	Increased blood flow
COMPRESSION	Decreased pain control	**A**NALGESIC	Increased pain control
ELEVATION	Incomplete healing	**T**REATMENT	Complete healing

Figure 3-1: RICE versus MEAT

THREE STAGES OF HEALING

	INFLAMMATORY	FIBROBLASTIC	MATURATION
Effect on blood	Increased blood flow	Formation of new blood vessels	New blood vessels mature
Symptoms	Swelling and pain increase	Swelling and pain subside	If tissue is strong, pain subsides
Physiology	Immune cells, called macrophages, remove damaged tissue	Immune cells, called fibroblasts, form new collagen	Increased density and diameter of collagen fibers occur if healing is not hindered
Length of time	Immediate response occurs for a week	Begins at day 2 or 3 after injury and continues for 6 weeks	Continues from day 42 until 18 months after injury

Figure 3-2: Three Stages of Healing After Soft Tissue Injury

Healing of an injured tissue, such as a ligament, progresses through a series of stages: inflammatory, fibroblastic, and maturation.[5-7] The inflammatory stage is characterized by an increase in blood flow, transporting healing immune cells to the area, often resulting in painful swelling. Swelling tells the body, especially the brain, that an area of the body has been injured. The immune system is activated to send immune cells, called polymorphonuclear cells, also known as "polys," to the injured area and remove the debris. *(See Figure 3-3.)* Other immune cells, including the monocytes, histocytes, and macrophage cells, assist in the cleanup. The macrophages and polys begin the process of phagocytosis, also called dinner, whereby they engulf and subsequently destroy debris and any other foreign matter in the body.

PROLOTHERAPY STIMULATES INFLAMMATION

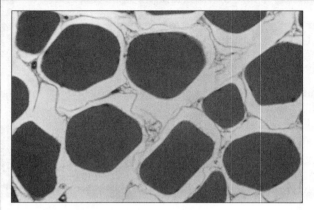

NORMAL MUSCLE TISSUE

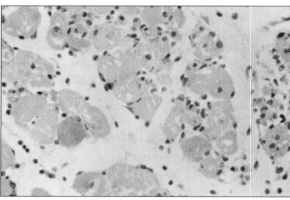

MUSCLE TISSUE 48 HOURS AFTER PROLOTHERAPY:
Injections with 12.5 percent Dextrose in 0.5 percent Xylocaine.

Notice the massive inflammatory reaction—the basis of Prolotherapy.

Slides prepared by Gale Bordon, M.D., from K. Dean Reeves, M.D. Used with permission.

Figure 3-3: Prolotherapy Stimulates Inflammation
Prolotherapy stimulates the natural healing mechanisms of the body via inflammation.

A day or two after the initial injury, the fibroblastic stage of healing begins. The body forms new blood vessels, a process called angiogenesis, because of factors released by the macrophage cells. Fibroblasts are formed from local cells or other immune cells in the blood. They are the carpenters of the body that form new collagen tissue, the building blocks of ligaments and tendons. Collagen is responsible for the strength of the ligament and tendon. The fibroblastic stage continues for approximately four to six weeks after the injury. Consequently, Prolotherapy treatments are typically administered every four to six weeks, allowing maximal time for ligament and tendon growth.[8]

The maturation phase of healing begins after the fibroblastic stage and may continue for 18 months after an injury. During this time the collagen fibers increase in density and diameter, resulting in increased strength.

NSAIDs versus Prolotherapy

	NSAIDs	PROLOTHERAPY
Proteoglycan Synthesis	Inhibited	Enhanced
Cartilage Healing	Inhibited	Enhanced
Progression of Arthritis	Enhanced	Inhibited
Fibroblast Proliferation	Inhibited	Enhanced
Muscle Repair	Inhibited	Enhanced
Tendon Strength	Inhibited	Enhanced
Ligament Healing	Inhibited	Enhanced
Overall Effect on Soft Tissue Healing	Inhibited	Enhanced

Figure 3-4: Comparison of the Effects of NSAIDs versus Prolotherapy on Soft Tissue Healing

The overall effect of NSAIDs on soft tissue healing is inhibition, whereas Prolotherapy is stimulation.

Anything that decreases inflammation is detrimental to the healing process of soft tissue injury. NSAIDs, for example, should only be prescribed when inflammation is the cause of the problem. In the case of soft tissue injury, inflammation is the cure for the problem. Thus, NSAIDs inhibit healing, whereas Prolotherapy enhances it. *(See Figure 3-4.)* Prolotherapy injections stimulate ligament and tendon tissue growth, which only occurs through the process of inflammation. Dr. Solomon was indeed right. Inflammation is the key to the treatment of human ailments. Those who suffer from chronic pain from conditions such as knee injuries have a choice: anti-inflame the pain to stay or inflame your pain away with Prolotherapy. ■

BIBLIOGRAPHY

1. Robbins, S. *Pathologic Basis of Disease.* Third Edition. Philadelphia, PA: W.B. Saunders. 1984, p. 40.
2. Greenfield, B. *Rehabilitation of the Knee: A Problem-Solving Approach.* Philadelphia, PA: F.A. Davis. 1993.
3. Woo, S. Injury and repair of the musculoskeletal soft tissues. *American Academy of Orthopaedic Surgeons.* 1987.
4. Mankin, H. Localization of tritiated thymidine in articular cartilage of rabbits inhibits growth in immature cartilage. *Journal of Bone and Joint Surgery.* 1962; 44A:682.
5. Robbins, S. *Pathologic Basis of Disease.* Third Edition. Philadelphia, PA: W.B. Saunders. 1984, p. 40.
6. Greenfield, B. *Rehabilitation of the Knee: A Problem-Solving Approach.* Philadelphia, PA: F.A. Davis Co.. 1993.
7. Woo, S. Injury and repair of the musculoskeletal soft tissues. *American Academy of Orthopaedic Surgeons.* 1987.
8. Benedetti, R. Clinical results of simultaneous adjacent interdigital neurectomy in the foot. *Foot and Ankle International.* 1996; 17:264-268.

CHAPTER 4

Prolotherapy Stimulates the Body to Repair Painful Areas

"...Prolotherapy is a method of injection treatment designed to strengthen 'the weld of disabled ligaments and tendons to bone by stimulating the production of new bone and fibrous cells.'..."
–George S. Hackett, M.D. • Father of Prolotherapy

WHAT IS PROLOTHERAPY IN SIMPLE TERMS?

It took Marion and me a while to figure out the best way to tell people about Prolotherapy. If fact, prior to our first national TV appearance for promoting *Prolo Your Pain Away!*, we took a media lesson from Dave Baum. He helps people with their presentations and gives them a behind-the-scenes look at television, radio, and print media. He said "Okay, tell me, what is Prolotherapy?" Our confident response, "It is an injection technique whereb..." Dave butts in..."Ooh, injections! No way! I am afraid of needles!" Then he reprimands us, "Come on, you have a three-minute spot on NBC, the host is going to talk for 60 seconds, and you have 120 seconds, if you're lucky, to explain everything about Prolotherapy. You better mention *Prolo Your Pain Away!*, you better make sure that the audience likes you, and you better wear a blue blazer with a light blue shirt..." We were overwhelmed. Talk about pressure. We thought college was tough!

Dave went on to tell us that when you mention "injections" right off the bat, you have lost a good number of people in your audience—people do not want to hear "injection"—no one likes injections! "Do you like injections?" he asked us. We had to admit we do not much care for injections either. With that in mind, Dave asked us again, "Okay, now what is Prolotherapy?" I (Ross) took a deep breath, confidently and boldly he proclaimed, "Prolotherapy is a treatment that strengthens ligaments and tendons..." Then Dave chimes in speaking like a nice southern older gentleman, "Hey Martha, this fella is talking about liniments. Is that the stuff you rub on your skin when your bursitis acts up?" The point was well taken. Too often medical people speak in medical language and expect everyone to understand them. Why should the average person know anything about ligaments and tendons? Many people know a lot about medicine and some probably do know about ligaments and tendons, but nothing can be assumed.

We spent the next 45 minutes coming up with the central message to answer the question "What is Prolotherapy?" Prolotherapy is a treatment that **stimulates the body to repair the painful area**. The average person watching TV, listening on the radio, or reading the newspaper or a magazine article completely understands this statement. Throughout this book, this central statement will be repeated. If you see us on TV or hear us on the radio, you will hear it there, too.

This is because Prolotherapy is the only treatment for someone with chronic pain or a chronic nagging sports injury that is generally strong enough to stimulate the body to repair the **exact** painful area.

Was the grueling eight-hour session with Dave Baum worth it? Well, two days later we flew to Los Angeles to the TV show taping. Immediately after the show, the host of *Doctor to Doctor* (TBN's second most popular show) Dr. Helen Pensati said, "This show is going to be on my all-time best show list." Dave Baum, you are the best!*

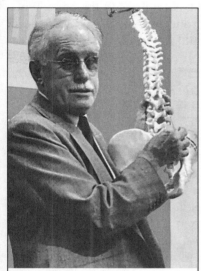

Figure 4-1:
George S. Hackett, M.D.
Demonstrating Prolotherapy at the AMA Convention in 1955.

GEORGE S. HACKETT, M.D.: DEFINITION OF PROLOTHERAPY

The official definition of Prolotherapy in *Webster's Third New International Dictionary* is "the rehabilitation of an incompetent structure, such as a ligament or tendon, by the induced proliferation of new cells."[1] The term was coined by George S. Hackett, M.D., in 1955. He describes Prolotherapy as follows: "The treatment consists of the injection of a solution within the relaxed ligament and tendon which will stimulate the production of new fibrous tissue and bone cells that will strengthen the weld of fibrous tissue and bone to stabilize the articulation (where the bone and ligament meet) and permanently eliminate the disability. To the treatment of proliferating new cells, I have applied the name *Prolotherapy* from the world 'Prolo' (Latin) meaning offspring; 'proliferate'—to produce new cells in rapid succession (Webster's Dictionary). My definition of Prolotherapy as applied medically in the treatment of skeletal disability is 'the rehabilitation of an incompetent structure by the generation of new cellular tissue.'"[2]

Dr. Hackett, after 20 years of seeing a lot of accident victims, arrived at the conclusion that injured ligaments were the primary cause of chronic pain. Injured tendons were the second most common cause. He referred to the weakness in the ligaments and tendons as laxity. His book is entitled *Ligament and Tendon Relaxation* (Skeletal Disability) *Treated by Prolotherapy* (Fibro-Osseous Proliferation).[2] "Fibro" is for fibrous and "osseous" stands for bone. Prolotherapy involves the injection of substances that cause stimulation at the fibrous tissue (ligaments and tendons) junction with the bone. The site where ligaments and tendons are typically injured is at their junction with the bone.

---

* Dave Baum Media Training Group • 7848 Kildare Avenue, Skokie, IL 60076 • 847-676-2155

Most things break down at a junction site because this is the weakest part of the structure. This is especially true in the weight-bearing joints. A good example of this is when the leg of a chair is wobbly or loose. This is usually due to a loose connection where the leg attaches to the seat of the chair. By tightening the attachment of the leg to the seat, the chair becomes more stable.

PROLOTHERAPY IS LIKE SPOT WELDING.

Dr. Hackett used the word "weld," which is a very accurate description of Prolotherapy. **Prolotherapy welds the ligaments and tendons to the bone**. When welding steel, the welder is applying a very hot probe or flame to melt two pieces of metal together. Two large pieces of metal would require welding many areas all along the long seam. Why do so many spots need to be welded? The reason is to make a stronger connection. If one area weakens in the future due to wear and tear, the others will hold the structure together.

This is the concept behind Prolotherapy. All of the injured tissue must be treated for sports injuries for chronic pain to be eliminated. People often ask, "Why do I have to receive so many shots?" I love to reply, "The more I give you, the more likely I am going to get at least one shot in the right place!" Okay, so my humor is not that funny. Maybe you just had to be there. The real reason so many injections are necessary at one visit is because Prolotherapy causes the proliferation of the weakened ligaments and tendons exactly where the injections are given. It is just like spot welding. It strengthens the exact spot where the weld or injection takes place. The more shots, the stronger the weld.

Dr. Hackett called Prolotherapy a treatment to permanently strengthen the weld of disabled ligaments and tendons to bone, by stimulating the production of new bone and fibrous tissue cells. So successful was Prolotherapy that he noted that the adoption of improved diagnosis and treatment by Prolotherapy of skeletal disability by orthopedic and neurological surgeons reduced spinal fusion operations by 95 percent.[2]

PROLOTHERAPY SUPPORTED IN THE LITERATURE

Dr. Hackett assumed that surgeons would readily learn the technique. The book reviewer for the *Journal of the American Medical Association* wrote in his review of Dr. Hackett's book, "An interesting and challenging book…the report of such a high incidence of recovery of the patients treated by the author should cause **all** physicians whose minds are not closed to new ideas to study the methods used and put them to the therapeutic test."[2] Another major medical journal, the *British Journal of Physical Medicine*, wrote, "I hope the book, *Ligament and Tendon Relaxation Treated by Prolotherapy*, will be widely read by orthopedic surgeons, especially those who are inclined to resort to surgery too rapidly. Here is a method which is not harmful and may well save a lot of laminectomies and save many patients from being trussed up in corsets."[2] Even state medical society journals were excited. For instance the *Ohio State Medical*

Journal wrote, "The book has been written so as to enable the reader to successfully carry out the diagnosis and treatment."[2] The American Medical Association was so excited about Prolotherapy that they let Dr. Hackett make presentations at their scientific exhibits several times in the 1950s. All of the above occurred in the late 1950s. *(See Appendix D, George S. Hackett AMA Presentations.)* The above confirms that Prolotherapy is a safe treatment that is easily learned, which not only treats, but also confirms the diagnosis and eliminates a lot of unnecessary surgeries. Why aren't all physicians, especially orthopedic surgeons and sports medicine physicians, doing it?

GUSTAV HEMWALL, M.D.

In 1955, Dr. Gustav Hemwall learned Prolotherapy from Dr. Hackett himself. He became so proficient at it that Dr. Hackett immediately began referring patients to Dr. Hemwall *(See Figure 4-3, Dr. Hackett Letter.)* In all of his many years of practice doing everything from delivering babies to surgery, Dr. Hemwall said that the most exciting thing for him in the practice of medicine was still Prolotherapy, because in doing the treatment unbelievable results were seen. Imagine that. Dr. Hemwall became a doctor in the 1930s, delivered babies, performed all kinds of surgery, saw antibiotics and modern medicines discovered, and what gave him the most reward? Seeing a disabled person, crippled over in pain, become completely pain-free. That is awesome to see! Anyone who knew Dr. Hemwall would concur that the man enjoyed giving shots, but more importantly he loved the hugs. Dr. Hemwall is very significant in the history of Prolotherapy because he was the main teacher of Prolotherapy from the late 1960's until the mid 1990's. I come into this picture because I was the doctor who took over the practice of Dr. Hemwall when he retired. *(See Figure 4-2.)*

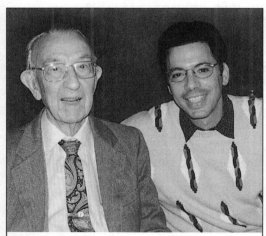

Figure 4-2
Dr. Hemwall and Dr. Hauser—the history and the future of Prolotherapy.

THE LIGAMENT REFERRAL PATTERNS

The chief principle of Prolotherapy is that it treats the root cause of chronic pain and sports injuries—ligament and tendon weakness. The chief symptom of ligament and/or tendon injury is pain. The pain is aggravated by activity when tension is placed upon the ligament or tendon and usually subsides when the tension is relieved with inactivity. Often the general activity of the athlete is curtailed because of the pain.

GEORGE S. HACKETT. M. D.
616 FIRST NATIONAL BANK BUILDING
CANTON 2. OHIO

Jan. 25, 1957

Mrs. Lloyd D. Anderson
315 South 12th Street
Albia, Iowa

Dear Mrs. Anderson:

In reply to your letter of the 21st,
I would suggest that you consult: -

Gustav A. Hemwall, M.D.
839 North Central Avenue
Chicago, Illinois.

Dr. Hemwall is the only man that I
know of in your part of the country who is
experienced with this technic of treatment.
He was out here on several occasions and was
instructed in the technic by me, and I can
recommend him highly.

As to whether your condition could
be benefitted by this procedure, it is
impossible to give you any answer without
first having examined you to determine your
disability.

If I can be of further service,
please feel free to call on me.

Sincerely,

George S. Hackett, M.D.

GSH/mak

Figure 4-3 Dr. Hackett's Letter

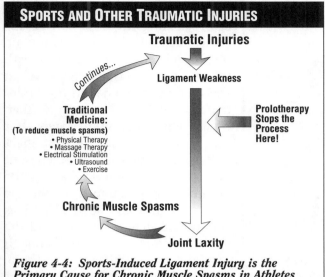

Figure 4-4: Sports-Induced Ligament Injury is the Primary Cause for Chronic Muscle Spasms in Athletes
Traditional Sports Medicine physiotherapy treatments often do not cure sports injuries because they do not get at the root cause—ligament weakness.

Severe pain from muscle spasm can occur from ligament and tendon weakness because the muscle is trying to stabilize the area. Chronic muscle spasms are almost always an indication of underlying ligament weakness. If the ligaments cannot stabilize the joint, the muscles contract to do it. *(See Figure 4-4.)* This is why treatments for sports and other traumatic injuries, such as physical therapy, electrical stimulation, and massage, often help to some degree, by relaxing the muscles, but do not cure the problem because the ligament laxity or weakness continues. Prolotherapy to strengthen the underlying joint and ligament permanently eliminates the pain.

The odd thing for an athlete is that sometimes the pain will totally dissipate between attacks. During this period a physician can still palpate the region and find the tender areas. When the tender areas are palpated, a female will squirm, but a male will jump because of his lower pain threshold. This is called a positive squirm and jump sign, respectively. *(See Figures 4-5 and 4-6.)*

What most athletic trainers, orthopedic surgeons, and physical therapists do not know is that ligaments can refer pain to a distant site. The more severe the injury, the more likely a referral pain pattern will exist. Dr. Hackett determined the referral patterns of the ligaments of the lower back, which refer to the legs, after giving 18,000 intraligamentous injections to 1656 patients over a period of 19 years.[2] *(See Ligament Referral Patterns in Figures 4-7 through 4-10.)* He determined that often sacroiliac ligament injury refers pain down the leg into the foot and is the reason for so-called "sciatica." Hip joint ligament injury refers pain down the leg into the big toe. Thus if a person has the respective ligament referral pattern, it helps the Prolotherapist determine which ligaments should be examined. The tender areas, as determined by a positive squirm or jump sign, are then injected. Ligament and/or tendon laxity (weakness) is one of the only conditions in which the diagnosis is confirmed before treatment and verified after each treatment. This one fact may be the reason for Prolotherapy's tremendously high success rate.

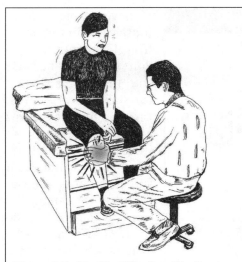

Figure 4-5: Positive "Squirm Sign"
Hitting the tender area by palpitation with the thumb or needle causes the woman to squirm, indicating the painful area has been located.

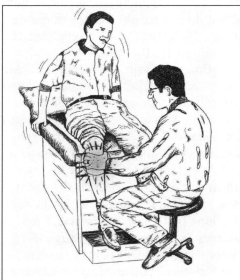

Figure 4-6: Positive "Jump Sign"
Hitting the tender area by palpitation with the thumb or needle causes men to **jump**. This is why Dr. Hemwall said he would rather treat 100 women than one man…

The treatment involves a physician palpating the exact site of the injury, reproducing the pain, and then confirming the diagnosis with the actual injections, because an anesthetic is contained in the Prolotherapy solution. The pain is then usually eliminated immediately after the treatment due to the effect of the anesthetic being injected right into the source of the pain—the fibro-osseous junction. Prolotherapy injections into all the tender areas will immediately eliminate all of the sharp pain and tenderness if enough solution of sufficient anesthetic strength is injected. Some people get so many injections that each injection can only contain a small amount of anesthetic solution (higher levels would be toxic). In such an instance, most of the pain will be immediately eliminated, but not all of it. Relieving the pain immediately after the Prolotherapy gives the athlete and the physician confidence that the injured structures have been treated.

RATE OF HEALING

Unfortunately for most, one treatment of Prolotherapy is not sufficient to cause enough growth of ligament and tendon tissue to permanently eliminate the chronic pain or sports injury. The typical young person requires about two or three treatments. We adults who are not lean, mean, fighting machines typically require anywhere from four to eight treatments. As you will learn, the inflammatory response typically occurs over a four to six week period, therefore most Prolotherapy physicians see patients for re-evaluation every four to six weeks. Athletes often do not have

HACKETT REFERRAL PATTERNS

Figure 4-7

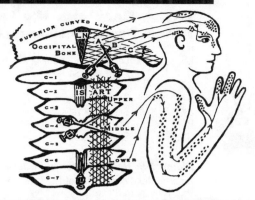

HEAD AND NECK REFERRAL PAIN PATTERNS
LIGAMENT AND TENDON RELAXATION

AREA OF WEAKNESS	REFERRAL PATTERN
OCCIPUT AREA A	FOREHEAD AND EYE
OCCIPUT AREA B	TEMPLE, EYEBROW AND NOSE
OCCIPUT AREA C	ABOVE THE EAR
CERVICAL VERTEBRAE #1-#3 (UPPER)	BACK OF NECK AND POSTERIOR SCAPULAR REGION (NOT SHOWN)
CERVICAL VERTEBRAE #4-#5 (MIDDLE)	LATERAL ARM AND FOREARM INTO THE THUMB, INDEX AND MIDDLE FINGER
CERVICAL VERTEBRAE #6-#7 (LOWER)	MEDIAL ARM AND FOREARM INTO THE LATERAL HAND, RING AND LITTLE FINGER

GLUTEUS MEDIUS MUSCLE
REFERRAL PATTERN
JANET TRAVELL, M.D.

THE GLUTEUS MEDIUS MUSCLE REFERS PAIN DOWN THE LATERAL LEG AND INTO THE BUTTOCK REGION.

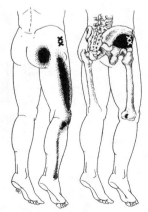

HIP LIGAMENT
REFERRAL PATTERN
GEORGE S. HACKETT, M.D.

THE HIP LIGAMENTS ALSO REFER PAIN DOWN THE LATERAL LEG AND INTO THE BUTTOCK REGION.

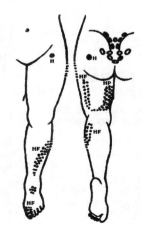

Figure 4-8: Comparison of Travell and Hackett Referral Patterns
Notice the similarities between the referral patterns.
Left: illustration: Travell—*Myofacial Pain and Disfucntion: The Trigger Point Manual*, Vol. 1, 2nd Ed., © Janet Travell, M.D. Used with permission.

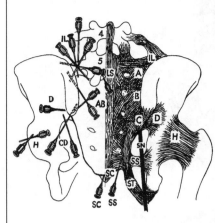

HACKETT REFERRAL PATTERNS

LOWER BACK AND HIP LIGAMENTS
TRIGGER POINTS OF LIGAMENTS

IL:	ILIOLUMBAR
LS:	LUMBOSACRAL—SUPRA AND INTERSPINUS
A, B, C, D:	POSTERIOR SACROILIAC
SS:	SACROSPINUS
ST:	SACROTUBERUS
SC:	SACROCOCCYGEAL
H:	HIP—ARTICULAR
SN:	SCIATIC NERVE

Figure 4-9: Hackett Referral Patterns
Ligamentous structures of the lower back and hip that refer pain down the lower leg. The illustration shows the trigger points of pain and the needles in position for confirmation of the diagnosis and for treatment of ligament relaxation of the lumbosacral and pelvic joints.

HACKETT REFERRAL PATTERNS

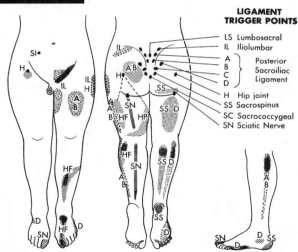

LIGAMENT TRIGGER POINTS

LS	Lumbosacral
IL	Iliolumbar
A B C D	Posterior Sacroiliac Ligament
H	Hip joint
SS	Sacrospinus
SC	Sacrococcygeal
SN	Sciatic Nerve

Figure 4-10

PAIN REFERRAL PATTERNS
FROM LUMBOSACRAL AND PELVIC JOINT LIGAMENTS

ABBREVIATION	LIGAMENT	REFERRAL PATTERN
IL:	ILIOLUMBAR	GROIN, TESTICLES, VAGINA, INNER THIGH
AB:	POSTERIOR SACROILIAC (UPPER ⅔ RDS)	BUTTOCK, THIGH, LEG (OUTER SURFACE)
D:	POSTERIOR SACROILIAC (LOWER OUTER FIBERS)	THIGH, LEG (OUTER CALF) FOOT (LATERAL TOES)— ACCOMPANIED BY SCIATICA
HP:	HIP—PELVIC ATTACHMENT	THIGH—POSTERIOR AND MEDIAL
HF:	HIP—FEMORAL ATTACHMENT	THIGH—POSTERIOR AND LATERAL LOWER LEG—ANTERIOR AND INTO THE BIG TOE AND 2ND TOE
SS:	SACROSPINUS & SACROTUBERUS	THIGH—POSTERIOR LOWER LEG—POSTERIOR TO THE HEEL
SN:	SCIATIC NERVE	CAN RADIATE PAIN DOWN THE LEG

six weeks to wait for their next treatment. The athlete will tell the doctor something along these lines, "Doctor, the PGA tour starts in six weeks. I need to be healed by that time." In such an instance, the athlete may be treated weekly or every other week.

There is usually a step-wise progression of healing after Prolotherapy for the person who receives Prolotherapy every four to six weeks. *(See Figure 4-11.)* As you know, the anesthetic in the solution used during Prolotherapy sessions often provides immediate pain relief. The pain relief may continue, after the effect of the anesthetic subsides, due to the stabilizing of the treated joints because of the inflammation caused by the Prolotherapy injections. This pain relief normally continues for a few weeks after each treatment.

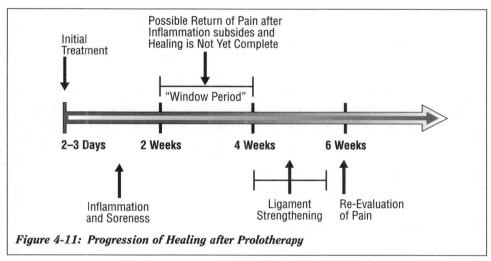

Figure 4-11: Progression of Healing after Prolotherapy

Between the second and fourth weeks, the initial stabilization induced by the Prolotherapy subsides, and because the initial growth of ligament tissue is not complete, some of the original pain may return during this "window period" of healing. The patient is typically seen for follow-up four to six weeks after the treatment so progress can be accurately assessed, avoiding evaluation during the "window period." Prolotherapy is performed every four to six weeks because most ligaments and tendons heal over this time frame.

As the healing progresses, the number of injections required per treatment usually decreases. The pain generally continues to diminish with each treatment until it is completely eliminated, often after four to eight sessions.

In some cases, athletes or other chronic pain patients will not experience pain relief after their first or second Prolotherapy treatment. This does not necessarily mean that the therapy is not working, but rather it is an indication that the ligaments and tendons are not yet strong enough to stabilize the joints. The amount of collagen growth required for stabilization of the joint is different for each person. A patient who experiences pain relief at rest, but not during activity requires further treatment to strengthen the area. If Prolotherapy treatments are continued, there is an excellent chance of achieving total pain relief with the resumption of all previous activities, including athletics.

For the rare person who feels no relief with the third treatment, I often do a nutritional assessment to see if there is something impairing the healing process. Some people want to do all of this on the first visit, which is often ideal because all aspects of healing can be initially addressed. Remember that Prolotherapy starts the healing process, the body grows the stronger tissue. The healthier the person, the more the tissue will be stimulated to grow with each treatment. If a person has a depressed immune system because of hormonal problems, nutritional deficiencies, or other medical problems (e.g., diabetes, etc.), these will decrease the body's ability to heal. Smoking and excessive drinking of alcohol have the same effect. This is where techniques like metabolic typing, nutritional counseling, and overall natural medicine care are encouraged.

Another option available to the Prolotherapist is to increase the strength of the Prolotherapy solution. This will cause an increase in the proliferant ability of the solution—hopefully causing the growth of more tissue with each treatment. A consequence of increasing the strength of the solution is that the athlete will have more pain immediately after the anesthetic wears off. Not all people have the resiliency to tolerate this increased pain. With the normal gentle Prolotherapy solutions, generally only a small amount of soreness is felt after the treatments. It feels similar to the achy sensation after raking leaves. Your back is stiff and sore, but it is a good kind of soreness.

DO THE INJECTIONS HURT?

In regards to pain we might as well answer the question you are thinking, "Do the injections hurt?" Of course. Okay, let's go on. Actually, the injections feel like you are getting pinched each time the needle goes into the skin. The only problem with this is that some people, especially the big 250-pound linebackers who get Prolotherapy, are, shall we say, "babies" during the treatment. We try to do all we can to help these people at Caring Medical and Rehabilitation Services. We give the patients Prolo-stress-balls to squeeze and hold the patients' hands during the treatments. For those athletes who are really sensitive to injections, pain medications and tranquilizers may be given, such as Vicodin and Xanax, prior to the injections. In really tough cases intravenous Demerol may be given as needed. About 90 percent of our patients typically receive Prolotherapy without any sedation or pain medications and do very well—especially the women. Women are tough. The big, large, muscular guys—well, they may need a little pampering.

PROLIFERANT SOLUTIONS (WHAT IS INJECTED)

Most of this information is derived from the writings of Allen R. Banks, Ph.D.[4] Proliferants used in Prolotherapy are basically substances that lead to new collagen formation. Collagen is the naturally occurring protein in the body that makes up ligaments and tendons. Prolotherapy solutions help strengthen these structures by initiating the first step in the wound-healing cascade, which is local inflammation. Once the inflammation has begun, fibroblasts are stimulated. These are the cells that make the collagen. New collagen is produced, making the ligaments and tendons stronger and tighter. The solutions vary in the mechanism by which they cause localized inflammation but, in general, they all act by causing localized tissue damage or irritation, which initiates the influx of inflammatory cells. The exception to this rule is sodium morrhuate, which probably acts more as a chemotactic (attraction) factor.[4]

OSMOTIC PROLIFERANTS (SOLUTIONS)

Osmotic proliferant solutions are the most commonly used proliferants and include dextrose and glycerin. These are injected and cause a higher osmotic (concentrated) gradient outside of the cells than inside of the cells. This causes cells to lose water and break. These broken cell particles stimulate an influx of inflammatory cells and initiate the wound-healing cascade to the specific area. Osmotic proliferants are water-soluble and thus, very safe. Being water-soluble means that whatever the body does not need is excreted out in the urine and is not stored in the fatty tissue of the body. Other proliferants in this class include the minerals zinc, calcium, and manganese. The minerals are also cofactors for various enzymes. For instance, manganese is needed for the enzyme superoxide dismutase, which helps the antioxidant status of the body. Since some people believe arthritis is from oxidative damage, some Prolotherapists, including those at Caring Medical and Rehabilitation Services, use manganese in the solution for arthritic patients.[5]

IRRITANTS

These are substances that are known to directly alter the proteins on the surfaces of the cells. They act by attaching themselves or their byproducts to the surfaces of the cells at the injection sites and they either damage the cells directly or render them reactive to the immune system. In either case, the immune cells are attracted to the area and start the immune response. The irritants that are used most commonly in Prolotherapy include dextrose, phenol, guaiacol, tannic acid, and plasma QU (quinine, urea). The Prolotherapy solution used in the two double-blinded studies was P2G, which included phenol, glycerin, and glucose. The author of this book uses an alkaline extract of the pitcher plant called Sarapin. The exact mechanism of how Sarapin relieves pain is unknown but is felt to be due to the ammonium sulfate concentrate in the extract of the plant.[6] It is plausible that this ammonium sulfate compound, or some yet unidentifiable biological agent in the pitcher plant, causes a gentle irritation which adds to the proliferant effect of the solution when Sarapin is added.

PARTICULATES

The most common particulate proliferant used is pumice flour. These small particles on the order of one micron, are notable for their ability to attract macrophages, which immediately phagocytize (eat up) the particles. Once the macrophages are at the injection site and ingesting pumice granules, they are actively secreting polypeptide growth factors, which ultimately result in collagen tissue growth.

CHEMOTACTICS

Chemotactics are proliferants that directly attract the immune cells to the injured area. Sodium morrhuate is thought to work in this way. Sodium morrhuate is the sodium salt of the fatty acid component derived from cod liver oil. Cold water fish oils are rich in polyunsaturated fatty acids, such as arachidonic acid. These compounds serve as the direct precursors to inflammation mediators. In this way, Sodium Morrhuate may directly attract the immune system to the area. Sodium morrhuate most resembles Sylnasol, one of the first proliferants ever used in Prolotherapy.

GROWTH FACTORS

Growth factors represent the future of Prolotherapy. As modern medicine makes advances in the regenerative mechanisms of the human body, many new growth factors are being discovered. Their effects are being tested as they directly stimulate the repair of various cells, organs, and diseases. Polypeptide growth factors act directly upon fibroblasts (which make collagen). Epidermal growth factor, insulin-like growth factors, fibroblast growth factors, and platelet-derived growth factors are now available for research and testing purposes. Physicians are already using Growth Hormone injections directly into joints to help regenerate cartilage. Many of these growth factors are available in homeopathic form to be taken orally during the Prolotherapy treatment course. As medical research continues, it is most assuredly certain that these growth factors will be incorporated into the technique of Prolotherapy.

THE FUTURE OF PROLIFERANT SOLUTIONS

We (Ross and Marion) attended the Medical conference in Dusseldorf, Germany, in October 1998 while on our European learning excursion studying with some of the world expert's on various techniques, including Neural Therapy. The Medical conference is the largest medical conference in the world. Over 110,000 people attended the conference to see some of the best and most innovative therapeutic and diagnostic information presented. Medical diagnostic testing, especially for soft tissue structures, is continually improving. It is now possible to determine bone density right in the doctor's office, without having to go to the hospital. The latest diagnostic technology for examining soft tissue injuries is using ultrasound. It is now possible to see most tendonitis, ligament sprains, or tears with ultrasound. Ultrasound is now being used in doctors' offices to actually see exactly where the needle is going. In the future, ligament sprains and tears will be commonly documented with radiography, but we suspect that even then the best diagnostic agent will remain the big "T"— the thumb. Nothing can ever top the fact that the thumb can totally and completely reproduce the pain. Ultrasound, MRI, or any other machine will never be able to do that.

There is no doubt that scientific documentation of the pathologic lesion will occur, where doctors doing Prolotherapy will use ultrasounds and other gadgets to help document the lesions being treated. Prolotherapists will use these gadgets, not because it helps the patient get better, but because it helps the patient get insurance reimbursement for the treatment. This is one of the reasons why health care costs are so high; someone has to pay for the expensive gadgets. This is one of the reasons Caring Medical has very few gadgets in the office. One of the gadgets that I (Ross) have is an electronic putting green, so I can play golf without ever leaving the office. I feels this makes him more well-rounded.

Future proliferants used in Prolotherapy will likely be the exact proliferants used by the human body to grow and repair connective tissue. Currently, physicians use such substances as dextrose (corn extract), sodium morrhuate (cod liver oil extract), Sarapin (pitcher plant extract), manganese, glucosamine, silica, pumice flour, zinc, glycerin, phenol, calcium, as well as various anesthetics in the Prolotherapy solution. These all have the effect of stimulating fibroblastic proliferation. These solutions ultimately increase the levels of the actual growth factors by which fibroblasts and chondrocytes divide and proliferate. It is these growth factors that actually cause the chondrocytes to regenerate cartilage and the fibroblasts to regenerate ligaments and tendons. It is these growth factors that will eventually be injected directly into the cartilage, ligaments, and tendons to proliferate the connective tissues.

Ligament research is being directed at the actual growth factors that stimulate ligament growth directly. Biomechanical studies of growth factor-treated ligament injuries have illustrated that transforming growth factor beta type 1 works to improve ligament healing, as shown by increased rupture force, stiffness, and breaking energy.[7] Other growth factors, including platelet-derived growth factor, basic fibroblast growth factor, and insulin-like growth factor type 1 have demonstrated properties that could also be helpful in healing ligament injuries.[8] Platelet-derived growth factor is a chemotactic agent for cells such as fibroblasts (attracts them to the area), and it also acts to increase the number of fibroblasts available to actively replicate.[9,10] Basic fibroblast growth factor, like platelet-derived growth factor, works chemotactically and by stimulating the proliferation of fibroblasts.[11] Insulin-like growth factor type 1, like platelet-derived growth factor, increases the number of fibroblasts available to actively replicate.[12] Insulin-like growth factor type 1, platelet-derived growth factor, and fibroblast growth factor have all been shown to enhance wound healing.[13, 14]

In one study done at the University of North Carolina School of Medicine, Department of Orthopedic Surgery, the researchers tested the hypothesis that injections of platelet-derived growth factor (PDGF) alone or in these combinations would increase the healing efficiency of ligaments:

● *PDGF plus Insulin-Like Growth Factor Type 1*
● *PDGF plus Basic Fibroblast Growth Factor*
● *Basic Fibroblast Growth Factor plus Insulin-Like Growth Factor Type 1*

This hypothesis was derived because of their effects on different parts of the cell replication cycle and their abilities to induce chemotaxis.[8] The study involved transecting the medial collateral ligaments of a Sprague-Dawley rat and then injecting one ligament with growth factor(s) and using the other side as a control. The rats were then sacrificed only 12 days later and the ligaments studied. Amazingly, in only 12 days ligaments receiving platelet-derived growth factor alone were 73 percent stronger than their contra-lateral internal controls. Stiffness increased by 94 percent and breaking energy by 101 percent over controls. *(See Figure 4-12.)* Ligaments treated with a combination of PDGF plus insulin-like growth factor type 1 and PDGF plus basic fibroblast growth factor also exhibited increases in rupture force, stiffness, and breaking energy over internal controls. The researchers concluded, "growth factors show great promise for improved healing... Growth factor studies in wound-chamber models suggest that platelet-derived growth factor initially produces a chemotactic stimulus. The migration of granulocytes, monocytes, and lymphocytes thus could be increased by the single application of growth factor at the time of injury. Once at the site of injury, these cells produce their own mitogenic and/or chemotactic factors, theoretically increasing fibro-blast numbers and eventually resulting in more collagen production at the injury site. The fact that platelet-derived growth factor can, with one application at the time of injury, increase the rupture force and stiffness of healing ligaments is promising." [8]

Growth factors are proteins that have been detected during the early phases of ligament healing and probably play the major role in the healing process. These proteins, among their many other functions, have been shown in

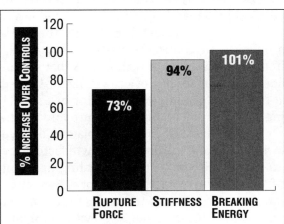

Figure 4-12: The Effect of Platelet Derived Growth Factors on Medial Collateral Ligament Healing
Rupture force, stiffness, and breaking energy increased by a remarkable 73%, 94%, and 101%, respectively, in only 12 days with just the addition of the growth factors. This is the future of sports medicine.

numerous studies to directly stimulate fibroblasts to proliferate, synthesize, and remodel the extracellular matrix (connective tissues).[15-18] Various researchers have shown that applications of these growth factors on injured ligaments can enhance the structural and mechanical properties of the healing ligament.[19,20] The various growth factors (especially platelet-derived growth factor, insulin-like growth factor type 1, and basic fibroblast growth factor) have been shown with one application to stimulate fibroblastic growth by a factor of 310 percent (3.1 times) and to increase the strength of the ligament-bone junctions by a factor of 240 percent (2.4 times) compared to non-treated ligament controls.[21,22] *(See Figure 4-13.)* These results are fantastic! Amazing! This will truly be the future of sports medicine.

PROLOTHERAPY CAUSES A RISE IN GROWTH FACTOR LEVELS

Much of the above research done on growth factors and their ability to stimulate ligament healing has been done in the past decade. The more research that is done on this topic the more promising the future looks for sports medicine. Recent research focusing on Prolotherapy has also looked at its effect on growth factors. The research found "nonsurgical repair of a lax anterior cruciate ligament (ACL) requires a rise in growth factors. Injection of a solution to stimulate a proliferative response (Prolotherapy) has typically relied upon stimulating the inflammatory cascade to create a rise in growth factors. However, hypertonic dextrose, up to 10 percent concentration, raises levels of basic fibroblast growth factor (bFGF), insulin growth factor-1 (IGF-1), platelet-derived growth factor (PDGF), and transforming growth factor alpha and beta (TGF-a & -b) without producing inflammation.[23] The studies done by K. Dean Reeves, M.D., at the University of Kansas Medical Center showed that for ACL ligament injury Prolotherapy caused a decrease in laxity of the ACL ligament by 33 percent. Pain with walking on level surfaces, uneven surfaces, or stairs, as well as subjective swelling and subjective looseness, decreased significantly because of the Prolotherapy injections.[23]

	Control	Platelet-Derived Growth Factor
Stiffness (N/mm)	22.4	24.4
Ultimate Load (N)	83.7	130.2
Energy Absorbed (J)	125	380
Ultimate Elongation (mm)	4.0	5.6

Figure 4-13: Structural Properties of the Femur-Medial Collateral Ligament Six Weeks after Injury

Ligaments injected with platelet-derived growth factor were thicker and stronger, as evidenced by the femur- medial collateral ligament—tibia complexes having ultimate load, energy absorbed to failure, and ultimate elongation values significantly greater than the control group.

Adapted from the American Journal of Sports Medicine, Vol. 26, No. 4, ©1998: The Effects of Platelet-Derived Growth Factor-BB on Healing of the Rabbit Medial Collateral Ligament—An In-Vivo Study, by Kevin A. Hildebrand, M.D., Savio L-Y Woo, Ph.D., David W. Smith, Christina R. Allen, M.D., Masataka Deie, M.D., Ph.D., Brian J. Taylor, M.S., and Christopher C. Schmidt, M.D.

The last study we would like to mention is perhaps the most encouraging in regard to the power of growth factors. Researchers at the Musculoskeletal Research Center at the University of Pittsburgh Medical Center analyzed the effects of individual growth factors on the proliferation of fibroblasts from the medial collateral and anterior cruciate ligaments of rabbits, in vitro, in order to identify growth factors that might enhance proliferation of fibroblasts and to compare the responses of the fibroblasts from the two ligaments to these growth factors.[24] The results of just this one study were unbelievable! *(See Figure 4-14.)* Through measurement of the uptake of (3H)-thymidine into DNA, fibroblasts from these ligaments, which had been treated with epidermal growth factor and basic fibroblast growth factor, were found to proliferate nearly eight times more than control fibroblasts. Additionally, the fibroblasts of both ligaments showed statistically significant increases in DNA uptake to acidic fibroblast growth factor and platelet-derived growth factor-BB. The authors justifiably concluded, "...this study demonstrated that growth factors can stimulate cell division in ligaments."[24]

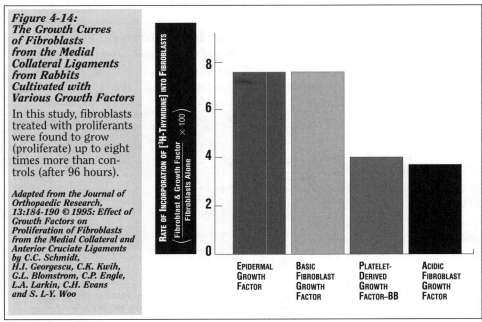

Figure 4-14:
The Growth Curves of Fibroblasts from the Medial Collateral Ligaments from Rabbits Cultivated with Various Growth Factors

In this study, fibroblasts treated with proliferants were found to grow (proliferate) up to eight times more than controls (after 96 hours).

Adapted from the Journal of Orthopaedic Research, 13:184-190 © 1995: Effect of Growth Factors on Proliferation of Fibroblasts from the Medial Collateral and Anterior Cruciate Ligaments by C.C. Schmidt, H.I. Georgescu, C.K. Kwih, G.L. Blomstrom, C.P. Engle, L.A. Larkin, C.H. Evans and S. L-Y. Woo

SUMMARY

The basic mechanism of Prolotherapy is simple. *(See Figure 4-15.)* A substance is injected, which leads to local inflammation. The localized inflammation triggers a wound-healing cascade, resulting in the deposition of new collagen. New collagen shrinks as it matures. The shrinking collagen tightens the ligament that was injected and makes it stronger. Prolotherapy has the potential of being 100 percent effective at eliminating sports injuries and chronic pain, but

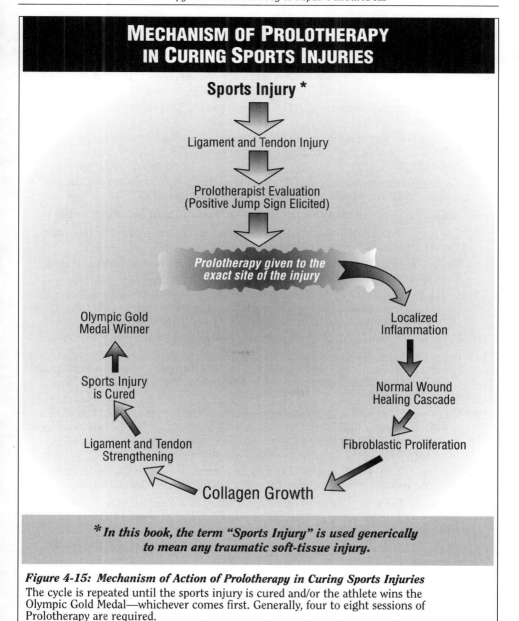

MECHANISM OF PROLOTHERAPY IN CURING SPORTS INJURIES

Sports Injury *

Ligament and Tendon Injury

Prolotherapist Evaluation
(Positive Jump Sign Elicited)

Prolotherapy given to the exact site of the injury

Localized Inflammation

Normal Wound Healing Cascade

Fibroblastic Proliferation

Collagen Growth

Ligament and Tendon Strengthening

Sports Injury is Cured

Olympic Gold Medal Winner

* In this book, the term "Sports Injury" is used generically to mean any traumatic soft-tissue injury.

Figure 4-15: Mechanism of Action of Prolotherapy in Curing Sports Injuries
The cycle is repeated until the sports injury is cured and/or the athlete wins the Olympic Gold Medal—whichever comes first. Generally, four to eight sessions of Prolotherapy are required.

depends upon the technique of the individual Prolotherapist. The most important aspect is injecting enough of the solution into the injured and weakened area. If this is done, the likelihood of success is excellent. ▪

59

BIBLIOGRAPHY

1. Babcock, P. et al. *Webster's Third New International Dictionary*. Springfield, MA: G. & C. Merriam Co. 1971, p. 1815.

2. Hackett, G. *Ligament and Tendon Relaxation Treated by Prolotherapy*. Third Edition. Springfield, IL: Charles C. Thomas, Publisher. 1958.

3. Personal correspondence with Dr. Paul Jordan via telephone, December 23. 1998.

4. Hemwall, G. Ligament and Tendon Relaxation Treated by Prolotherapy. Fifth Edition. Oak Park, IL: Beulah Land Press. 1999, Chapter 13, pp. 287-295, by Banks, A.

5. Personal correspondence with Thomas Hesselink, M.D., secretary of the International Bio-Oxidative Medicine Association, July 1997.

6. High Chemical Company brochure entitled *Sarapin* sent to author in 1994.

7. Conti, N. The effect of exogenous growth factors on the healing of ligaments. Trans. Orthop. Res. Soc. 1993; 18:60.

8. Letson, A. The effect of combinations of growth factors on ligament healing. *Clinical Orthopaedics and Related Research*. 1994; 308:207-212.

9. Chen, Y. Altered cell cycle responses to insulin-like growth factor 1, but not platelet-derived growth factor and epidermal growth factor, in senescing human fibroblasts. *Journal of Cell Physiology*. 1990; 144:18-25.

10. Ross, R. The biology of platelet-derived growth factor. *Cell*. 1986; 46:155-169.

11. Gospodarowicz, D. Molecular and biological characterization of fibroblast growth factor, an angiogenic factor, which also controls the proliferation and differentiation of mesoderm and neuroectoderm derived cells. *Cell Differ*. 1986; 19:1-17.

12. Van Wyk, J. Paracrine, and autocrine effects of the somatomedins/insulin-like growth factors. In Isaksson, O. (ed.) Growth Hormone—Basic Clinical Aspects: *Proceedings of the First Nordisk Insulin Symposium*. Stockholm, Sweden. June/July, New York, Elsevier Science Publishers. 1987, 337-354.

13. Greenhalgh, D. PDGF and FGF stimulate wound healing in the genetically diabetic mouse. *American Journal of Pathology*. 1990; 136:1235-1246.

14. Lynch, S. The effects of short-term application of a combination of platelet-derived and insulin-like growth factors on periodontal wound healing. J. *Periodontol*. 1991; 62:458-467.

15. Clark, R. Cutaneous tissue repair: basic biologic considerations. *American Academy of Dermatology*. 1985; 13:701-725.

16. Hudson-Goodman, P. Wound repair and the potential use of growth factors. *Heart and Lung*. 1990; 19:379-384.

17. Lepisto, J. Effects of homodimeric isoforms of platelet-derived growth factor on wound healing in rats. *Journal of Surgical Research*. 1992; 53:596-601.

18. McGee, G. Recombinant basic fibroblast growth factor accelerates wound healing. *Journal of Surgical Research*. 1988; 45:145-153.

19. Batten, M. The influence of various doses of platelet-derived growth factor on ligament healing. *Trans. Ors*. 1995; 20:37.

20. Conti, N. The effect of exogenous growth factors on healing of ligaments. *Trans. Ors*. 1993; 18:60.

21. Scherping, S. Effect of growth factors on the proliferation of ligament fibroblasts from skeletally mature rabbits. *Connective Tissue Research.* 1997; 36:1-8.

22. Hildebrand, K. The effects of platelet-derived growth factor-BB on healing of the rabbit medial collateral ligament. *American Journal of Sports Medicine.* 1998; 26:549-554.

23. Reeves, D. Prospective randomized double-blind treatment comparison study of the effects of interarticular injection of hypertonic dextrose/xylocaine/benzyl alcohol solution versus hypotonic xylocaine/benzyl alcohol solution on laxity of the anterior cruciate ligament. *Abstract. Archives of Physical Medicine and Rehabilitation.* 1998; 79:1149.

24. Schmidt, C. Effect of growth factors on the proliferation of fibroblasts from the medial collateral and anterior cruciate ligaments. *Journal of Orthopedic Research.* 1995; 13:184-190.

CHAPTER 5

Prolotherapy to Stop the Arthritic Process

There are so many older athletes with arthritis in the knees, I want to make sure you get the message. If an athlete does not heal the cartilage, meniscus, ligament, or tendon injury when it occurs, he/she is just one more step closer to developing symptomatic arthritis. There is no reason for an athlete to get arthritis, when a treatment like Prolotherapy is available. Prolotherapy stops the arthritic process because it strengthens the joint, thus ending the need for the knee and other joints to grow bone or form bone spurs.

The key to stopping the arthritic process is keeping the articular cartilage healthy. The ends of the knee bones are lined with articular cartilage. This amazing structure, which is only one-eighth to one half-inch thick, works to distribute the load of each step and minimizes peak stresses by deforming and regaining its previous shape. Articular cartilage is also remarkable in that, once formed, it remains unchanged for many years unless due to injury or illness. It has a very low metabolic rate and lacks blood vessels as well as nerves. Under normal circumstances, cartilage cells (chondrocytes) in an adult rarely, if ever, divide. The nutrition required by these cells to stay alive is derived from the joint fluid. For the cartilage to remain healthy it must be regularly subjected to weight-bearing exercise.[1] Once injured, the articular cartilage makes only a very small attempt to repair itself. When a knee is examined one year after cartilage injury, it is virtually unchanged from 24 hours after the injury![2] That is— without Prolotherapy, of course!

Surgical solutions to damaged articular cartilage rely on "shaving" the cartilage or punching holes in the bone. These options should be considered carefully before a decision to proceed is made. The long-term results are guarded because of the arthritis risk, and the short-term results are average at best. Cartilage-shaving surgery is done frequently but its success has not been proven. In fact, one study found that shaving damaged articular cartilage did not restore a good surface, but rather caused increased shredding of the surface and death of the cartilage cells![3] The treatment by drilling holes has very unpredictable results. The bottom line is that surgery is typically not a good choice for helping to heal an injury to the articular cartilage.

Prolotherapy injections provide what the knee joint lining needs to heal. What it needs is a strong stimulus to heal! There is experimental and clinical evidence that saline irrigation or enzyme irrigation of the joint stimulates a repair.[4] That is, Prolotherapy very likely stimulates stem cells from other areas of the joint to migrate into the injured area. These stem cells change their form slightly and begin to make cartilage and other proteins that are needed for knee cartilage repair. With three to four series of injections, spaced a few weeks apart, pain from injury to the articular cartilage can be improved with Prolotherapy and activities restored! Prolotherapy, in my experience, has been the only treatment I have seen to effectively stimulate articular cartilage growth.

MENISCUS

A common injury to the knee is the torn meniscus, or cartilage. This often happens to young people who are active in sports. Most cartilage or meniscal injuries, however, occur during everyday situations, such as rising from a chair or catching your heel while descending stairs. This is because the mechanism of injury can be as simple as getting your foot caught on something while your knee twists. If your knee easily twists during activity while your foot is stationary, you are more likely to sustain a meniscal injury.

The athlete is especially prone to meniscus injuries. This is particularly true if the sport involves running and pivoting, such as in tennis and basketball. The meniscus is quite vulnerable to rotational stresses. The medial meniscus on the inner side of the knee is injured much more frequently, than the lateral meniscus on the outside of the knee, due to its stronger attachment to the medial collateral ligament and joint capsule. Men sustain three times as many meniscus injuries as women.[5] This most likely relates to the fact that men participate in more violent sports, such as football, rugby, and hockey, where many of these injuries occur.

The history of a torn meniscus is characteristic: a locking with the knee bent followed by unlocking by shaking the leg. These injuries almost always occur between the ages of 16 to 30. The knee hurts when fully bending it. Athletes can tell which side of the knee is hurt indicating medial or lateral meniscus injury.

The meniscus has several important functions in the knee. Perhaps its most important function is that it distributes the weight over a greater surface area. This helps prevent compression injuries from forces exerted through the knee. Its second function is that of a shock absorber. It is estimated that the intact meniscus absorbs up to 20 percent of the force of impact.[6] The meniscus also adds to the stability of the knee. This function is minor in an otherwise intact knee. If one or more of the major knee ligaments are injured, then its stabilizing function becomes more important, making it even more vital to preserve the meniscus.[7]

If the anterior cruciate ligament (ACL) is torn, then the meniscus, if it was not injured at the same time, is very likely to begin degenerative changes. This is because an ACL-deficient knee is generally unstable and needs Prolotherapy. The meniscus absorbs the forces caused by the instability for a time. When its time is up and it starts fatiguing, the arthritic process of the knee goes into high gear. Once the meniscus cannot bear the pressure, the articular cartilage must carry more of the load forces. Eventually it becomes deteriorated and the person starts losing motion of the knee and limiting activities. This is why meniscus preservation, not shaving, needs to become a movement in America. We want to preserve everything—forests, sea turtles, foods, why not meniscus? If the torn ACL is not repaired and the meniscus is repaired, a re-tear of the meniscus occurs in up to 46 percent of cases![8] In animal models these bad changes to the meniscus begin within a week after surgically cutting the ACL.[9] The moral of the story is that ligament weakness in only one ligament can cause the downfall and deterioration of everything else in the joint. Each individual ligament is important. As previously discussed, bracing and taping cannot replace even one weakened, stretched-out knee ligament. That particular injured ligament must be proliferated with Prolotherapy and made whole again. This is the only way to truly repair a joint.

Surgical removal of an injured meniscus is unfortunately often recommended for many athletes. While this is sometimes necessary, Prolotherapists urge athletes to give serious consideration to the facts before going under the knife. There is an overall complication rate for arthroscopic meniscal repair of 18 percent, with a staggering 29 percent complication rate if you happen to be a female athlete.[10] Removal of the meniscus has been clearly shown to cause degenerative arthritis of the knee and associated pain.[11] Osteoarthritis should be expected in up to 70 percent of cases after total meniscectomy.[12] The amount of knee degeneration is **directly proportional** to the amount of meniscus removed.[13] Other complications include infection, popliteal nerve injury, or blood vessel injury.[14]

One of the most troubling complications is dubbed "arthrofibrosis." This means a painful joint that is stiff and limited in its movement. It occurs in up to 10 percent of meniscal repairs when ACL reconstructive surgery is performed at the same time and in six percent when performed on an ACL-deficient knee without reconstruction.[15] The scary fact is that sometimes the arthrofibrosis cannot be helped, even with physiotherapy, and the person ends up with a loss of motion because of it. Generally, with ACL reconstruction the rehabilitation course is brutal, lasting months and months. For the athlete playing for a college or professional team, Prolotherapy makes a lot more sense, because the recovery period is much shorter. Any athlete contemplating a surgical procedure of the knee should consult a Prolotherapist for a second opinion. Your athletic career could depend on it.

In the intact knee the weight is distributed over approximately six square centimeters. When the medial meniscus is removed, the same weight is now distributed over as little as 30 percent of the original structure![16] This means that higher pressure is focused over a smaller area of the knee, leading to greatly increased stress on the knee and injury to the affected parts that take up the slack! The parts of the knee that are brutalized when the meniscus is removed are the collateral and cruciate ligaments, and the articular cartilage. When these go, the only remaining event that can happen to stabilize the knee is arthritis. This is why early interventional Prolotherapy, before osteoarthritis begins, is a good idea. *(See Figure 5-1.)* At least 50 percent of the load is

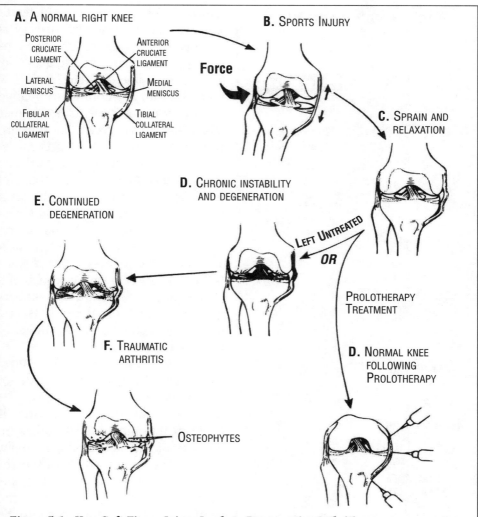

A. A NORMAL RIGHT KNEE

POSTERIOR
CRUCIATE
LIGAMENT

ANTERIOR
CRUCIATE
LIGAMENT

LATERAL
MENISCUS

MEDIAL
MENISCUS

FIBULAR
COLLATERAL
LIGAMENT

TIBIAL
COLLATERAL
LIGAMENT

B. SPORTS INJURY

Force

C. SPRAIN AND
RELAXATION

D. CHRONIC INSTABILITY
AND DEGENERATION

E. CONTINUED
DEGENERATION

LEFT UNTREATED

OR

PROLOTHERAPY
TREATMENT

F. TRAUMATIC
ARTHRITIS

D. NORMAL KNEE
FOLLOWING
PROLOTHERAPY

OSTEOPHYTES

Figure 5-1: How Soft Tissue Injury Leads to Degenerative Arthritis
Ligaments become sprained following trauma. When healing does not occur, the ligaments
become relaxed, resulting in chronic instability and degeneration from meniscal and
articular cartilage degeneration. When left untreated, post-traumatic "arthritis" or
degenerative osteoarthritis follows. This degenerative process can be prevented with
appropriate intervention through Prolotherapy.

carried by the meniscus with the knee straight and 85 percent with the knee
bent![17] As you can see, it is important to retain this structure in your knee for
as long as you can!

Sports are the overwhelming cause (82 percent) of meniscus and ACL injury
occurring together. In one study, when 177 meniscus injuries were treated surgically, the surgery failed in 36 percent, had partial healing in 38 percent, and a
full 20 percent had repeat arthroscopy within the three and a half year

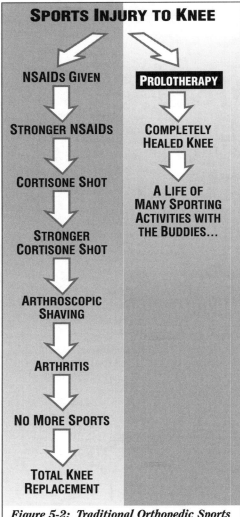

SPORTS INJURY TO KNEE

Figure 5-2: Traditional Orthopedic Sports Medicine vs. Prolotherapy
One path leads to a total knee replacement. The other leads to a totally normal knee—which would you rather have?

follow-up.[18] It is time for athletes to wake up and realize that surgery is not a panacea. It rarely cures the athletes' problems, and, at best, generally gives only temporary relief for a few years. Go into any chronic pain clinic and many of the patients are former athletes who have received a substantial amount of routine orthopedic care, including surgeries, cortisone shots, and NSAIDs. For the athlete of today, the choice is stay on the train that leads to joint replacement surgery by taking the NSAIDs and getting cortisone shots, or get Prolotherapy and stop the process. *(See Figure 5-2.)* It does not seem like much of a choice. But why then are the numbers of arthroscopies, cortisone shots, and knee replacements continuing to escalate in this country?

Back to the meniscus...the central two-thirds of the meniscus does not have a blood supply of its own.[2, 19] It receives its nutrition by "soaking" it up from the joint fluid it bathes in. Because of the lack of blood supply, this tissue does not heal back together, like a cut in the skin does, for example. Large, painful tears of the central meniscus often need to be treated surgically, but many physicians who utilize Prolotherapy have helped plenty of these "you must have surgery" cases. Prolotherapy can stimulate any soft tissue injury to heal. Prior to having meniscus removal surgery, it is definitely best to try to strengthen the meniscus with Prolotherapy!

LATERAL MENISCUS: CASE HISTORY

*Darrell is a 37 year old police officer. While snowboarding, he put his foot down and twisted his left knee. He had episodes of locking and painful popping

---

* *This chapter was written with the assistance of Rodney Van Pelt, M.D., of Ukiah, California. Find his office information and that of other Prolotherapists around the country at www.getprolo.com.*

associated with swelling and pain. Darrell's worst episode happened the day prior to his first visit to me. He could barely walk. I withdrew over one quarter cup of fluid from his knee and injected Prolotherapy solution into the joint. After drawing the fluid out two more times, I treated his lateral meniscus six times with Prolotherapy. After this he returned to both winter and summer sports and unrestricted police duties.

Swelling in a joint typically means that a structure inside the joint is injured, usually in the knee this is a cruciate ligament or meniscus. Either way, the best treatment is Prolotherapy.

Prolotherapy can effectively treat many meniscus injuries, especially those in the outer rim. The blood supply to the meniscus nourishes this outer rim and allows for easier healing. Unfortunately, only 15 to 20 percent of meniscus injuries occur in this outer third.[20] Studies have shown that the central two-thirds of the meniscus is capable of repair using the blood vessels from the joint lining (synovium) and the meniscus itself. It has been demonstrated that the cells of the meniscus can and do heal when exposed to certain growth stimulating factors.[21] Prolotherapy provides this stimulation to heal. This is why many athletes suffer-ing from the pain and disability of a torn meniscus are sucessfully treated by Prolotherapy instead of the much riskier surgeries.

THE CORONARY LIGAMENTS

The coronary ligaments hold the meniscus to the tibial plateau around the outside edge of the meniscus. Prolotherapy can strengthen these small but important ligaments and tack the cartilage back down and stimulate the regeneration of a peripheral tear. This allows the athlete to retain this very important piece of the knee! Every piece of the knee has a purpose, ordained by God.

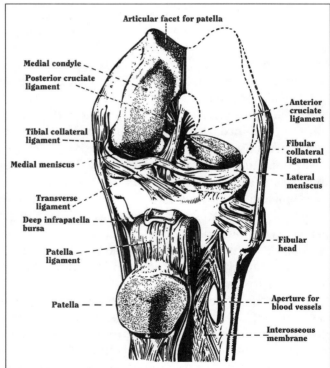

Articular facet for patella

Medial condyle

Posterior cruciate ligament

Tibial collateral ligament

Medial meniscus

Transverse ligament

Deep infrapatella bursa

Patella ligament

Patella

Anterior cruciate ligament

Fibular collateral ligament

Lateral meniscus

Fibular head

Aperture for blood vessels

Interosseous membrane

Figure 5-3: Anterior View of the Knee
The large cruciate ligaments inside the knee are the main stabilizers of the knee. Injury to these ligaments puts a tremendous strain on the remaining knee structures and accelerates the degenerative process.

God put the coronary ligaments in there for a purpose. If they are cut away, it will have an effect on the stability of the knee. This is why it is best to see a Prolotherapist when soft tissue is injured, even those as small as the coronary ligaments.

CRUCIATE LIGAMENTS

These are the deepest ligaments of the knee. They are approximately two inches long and primarily give the knee its anterior/posterior stability. *(See Figure 5-3.)* There are in the neighborhood of 200,000 ACL injuries each year.[22] These are one of the best publicized of knee injuries. There is actually a very good reason for this. While cruciate ligament tears are not the most common knee injury, they very commonly do not heal well. The blood supply is from within the ligament itself, not from around it, and therefore when the ligament is torn, the blood supply is commonly disrupted during the injury.[23] The cruciate ligament is unique in that it is inside the joint yet outside the synovial lining of the joint. This is possible because the capsule of the joint makes a kind of tube around both the anterior and posterior cruciate. They are not bathed in the joint fluid.

The anterior cruciate is frequently injured during sports such as football, soccer, and basketball. The most common cause of isolated ACL injury is a deceleration, cutting movement. When an athlete is struck by another player from behind and the outside, the ACL and medial collateral ligament (MCL) may both be injured. Injury is often accompanied by an audible "pop" usually with, and occasionally without, pain. If this injury occurs while bearing weight on the knee, the meniscus is regularly affected as well. The length and weight of downhill skis combined with failure of the bindings to release during a fall are a common cause of this type of injury during skiing, despite improved equipment.[24]

In one study the investigators looked at what happens if you do physical therapy and external bracing to treat a transected ACL. The results were dismal, even one and a half years after injury. There were a total of 32 percent who did "good" or "excellent," with a staggering 54 percent who did poorly! Thirty-five percent went ahead and had surgical reconstruction during the follow-up period.[25] ACL injuries need to be taken very seriously. The athlete with an ACL tear needs to seriously consider Prolotherapy. ACL-deficient knees are notoriously arthritis-provoking.

It is of the utmost importance to repair an injured cruciate ligament, especially ACLs.[26] On this point surgeons and Prolotherapists agree. PCL injuries do not seem to cause the long-term problems that ACLs cause. The only difference is how you repair it. If the ACL is completely torn, surgery is needed. For everything else, Prolotherapy should be instituted. Prolotherapy can definitely tighten up loose knees as long as the two ends of the ligament are still attached. Untreated, relaxed, or torn ACLs have clearly been shown to lead to degeneration of the meniscus and eventual degenerative arthritis.[27] Whereas treatment of the ACL seems to save the meniscus and preserve the joint from osteoarthritis.[28]

The posterior cruciate ligament (PCL) is also about two inches long. It limits backward motion of the tibia, the large bone just below the knee. It is uncommon to injure the PCL during sports. More commonly, it is injured during a motor vehicle accident when the knees hit the dashboard. A person who sustains a PCL injury without other associated ligament disruption will probably remain symptom free.[29] If pain does occur, Prolotherapy to the two attachments of the PCL inside the knee is effective at tightening these ligaments.

MRI scans are quite inaccurate at diagnosing cruciate ligament injury. They are not as accurate as one would think in differentiating between a complete tear and a partial tear.[30] I have had plenty of occasions where the MRI showed extensive knee damage and Prolotherapy completely relieved the pain. Obviously, the more extensive injuries in and around the knee require more Prolotherapy injections per visit, and often an increased number of visits. Ultimately, the athlete who chooses Prolotherapy is saying, "I want the problems fixed. How is the doctor giving me a cortisone shot going to fix the problem?" That is a sure way to keep an orthopedist quiet. Just ask that question.

Of course, surgery is repeatedly recommended for torn cruciate ligaments. Orthopedic surgeons desire to perform surgery for those cases where the football player hears a "pop" during a tackle. This is the reason why orthopedic surgeons are the team physicians: to operate on all the "pops." For anything except complete rupture (grade 3 injury) of the anterior cruciate ligament, avoid surgery if possible. The fact that there are so many ways to perform the surgery is an indication that there is no one excellent method. The repair of a transected cruciate ligament was successful in only two-thirds of 175 patients who were treated surgically, when followed up one to eight years later.[31] There is a better way and that way is Prolotherapy.

The complications of orthopedic surgery are significant and frequent. Most are outlined in the section on arthroscopy. The ligament grafts are profoundly weakened about eight weeks after surgery. At this time their strength is about 10 percent of its initial strength! It is only 50 percent of initial strength after one year. In two to three years the grafts are at their strongest, and then, less than their initial strength.[32] Compare this to one study where ligament strength was measured after a six-week period of doing Prolotherapy on knee ligaments. The results showed that in every case Prolotherapy increased ligamentous mass, thickness, and cross-sectional area as well as the ligament strength. Prolotherapy in a six-week period increased ligament mass by 44 percent, ligament thickness by 27 percent, and the ligament-bone junction strength by 28 percent.[33] There are other techniques for ACL problems, including artificial grafts. These artificial grafts (e.g., Gortex) lead to particularly poor results with very high complications![34, 35] Arthrofibrosis (a scarred, painful, stiff, knee with limited use) followed arthroscopic ACL reconstruction in 10 percent of the cases, when associated with the repair of a torn meniscus![36]

In an Australian study, patients were followed up after 7.4 years. Fifty-seven percent had pain on exertion. There was an overall significant deterioration of the anterior-posterior stability of the knee, indicating a failure of the ligament graft integrity with time.[37] In another study of patients followed for two to seven years after surgery, seven percent of the grafts failed and another 26 percent had only "fair" results.[38]

The truly phenomenal news is that Prolotherapy has been shown to stimulate healing in torn cruciate ligaments! The main evidence for this are the many athletes already healed by Prolotherapy. In a small study of athletes who had torn the cruciate ligaments, the knees were examined with a commercially-available computerized instrument, called an electrogoniometer, before and after Prolotherapy to their knees. The results were wonderful! The joint looseness was significantly decreased and the pain was markedly reduced or eliminated. They returned to a higher level of functioning, many returning to sports.[39] Even more impressive were the results of a double-blind placebo-controlled study of dextrose Prolotherapy for knee osteoarthritis with and without ACL laxity, performed by K. Dean Reeves, M.D. The study participants had six months or more of pain, along with either grade 2 or more joint narrowing or grade 2 or more osteophytic change in any knee compartment. A total of 38 knees were completely void of cartilage, radiographically, in at least one compartment. The study involved the injection of a dextrose Prolotherapy solution, bimonthly, comparing it to a control solution into 111 knees in 68 patients with osteoarthritis. The results showed that at 12 months, after six injections, the dextrose-treated knees improved in pain (44% decrease), swelling complaints (63% decrease), knee buckling frequency (85% decrease), and in flexion range (14 degree increase). Analysis of blinded radiographic readings of 0- and 12-month films revealed stability of all radiographic variables with two variables improving with statistical significance (lateral patellofemoral cartilage thickness and distal femur width in millimeter, both of which signify cartilage growth). Knees with ACL laxity showed statistically significant improvements in pain, swelling, joint flexion, and joint laxity. Amazingly, eight out of the 13 dextrose-treated knees with ACL laxity were no longer lax at the conclusion of one year.[40] These results were with only one Prolotherapy injection into the knee joints at each session. In other words, the ACL ligament attachments were not treated separately, which is routinely done during Prolotherapy for ACL laxity. Imagine what the results would be like if the ACL itself was treated! Yes, the athlete has a choice—Prolotherapy or surgery. The choice should be an easy one, especially if you see what surgery involves. *(See Figures 5-4a and 5-4b.)*

When Prolotherapy is given, the joint stability is restored and painless function returns! Because of the ligaments' location outside the capsule, these injections must be directed specifically at the ligament attachments to bone at all four ends of the cruciates, if they are both injured. A simple injection into the joint will not do the same thing, although this may be needed as well if arthritis is

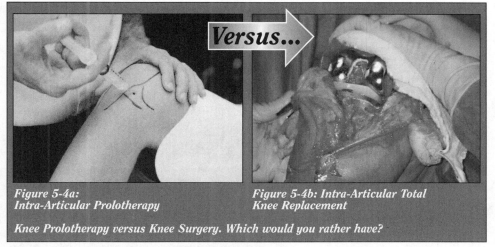

Figure 5-4a:
Intra-Articular Prolotherapy

Figure 5-4b: Intra-Articular Total
Knee Replacement

Knee Prolotherapy versus Knee Surgery. Which would you rather have?

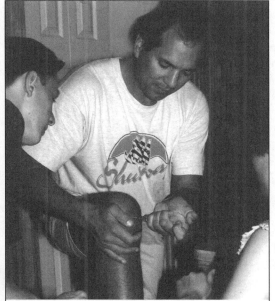

Figure 5-5: Dr. Rodney Van Pelt takes the phrase, "Physician, heal thyself" very seriously.

present from the injury. Prolotherapy is a simple solution for a myriad of seemingly complex knee problems. They all involve injury to the soft tissues of the knee (meniscus, cartilage, ligaments, or tendons) at their root cause. Since Prolotherapy is the only treatment that specifically regrows soft tissues at the exact site of injury, it is effective for the vast majority of knee conditions in athletes. *(See Figure 5-5.)*

ANTERIOR CRUCIATE: CASE HISTORY

Marion, a 15 year old basketball player, was the star of her team. She was high on life, until the day when another player fell on the back of her leg, when they were both going up for a rebound. She felt immediate pain, but continued to play the rest of the game. After the game her knee was painful and swollen. She limped around for a few days and it seemed to improve. Each time she played it would swell and hurt to where she needed to be pulled from the game.

Marion had torn her anterior cruciate ligament. Her knee was drained and she was given NSAIDs, which did nothing to get rid of her pain. She even considered surgery, but came to see me instead. She was in a great hurry to begin the season in 10 weeks, so she received Prolotherapy injections to the anterior cruciate ligaments of the injured knee once each week for five weeks. She allowed it to heal. She returned for the next season and, despite the lack of pre-season training, she went on to be a leading scorer—to her and her teammates' delight. Prolotherapy does indeed regenerate torn cruciate ligaments and, as a consequence, it allows people like Marion to get right back into their sporting activities without some prolonged rehabilitation program that is typically needed for knee ACL injuries. Is it any wonder why athletes from around the country are eagerly getting their sports injuries Prolo'ed away?

SUMMARY

Prolotherapy is useful for a wide range of sports knee injuries and is a much better option than cortisone shots, arthroscopy, and especially surgery. In many cases it can save the athlete from the risks associated with surgery, the long rehabilitation period after surgery, and the failures of surgery. Athletes often end up with arthritic knees, not because they exercised too much, but because their original knee injuries were not completely healed. This is often because athletes are given the RICE protocol with anti-inflammatories to decrease their pain. If this does not work, cortisone shots, arthroscopy, and other surgical recommendations are soon to follow. These are definitely decreasing the healing. Athletes are encouraged to use the MEAT protocol along with specific physiotherapy, and if needed, Prolotherapy after an injury. Prolotherapy is effective for the myriad of knee injuries, because all of them involve injuries to the soft tissue structures (meniscus, articular cartilage, tendons, and ligaments). With Prolotherapy the athlete heals sports injuries permanently, naturally, and safely! I thank our Creator for the wonderful gift of healing and for Prolotherapy that can stimulate that healing. ■

BIBLIOGRAPHY

1. Woo, S. Injury and repair of the musculoskeletal soft tissues. Park Ridge, IL: *American Academy of Orthopaedic Surgeons*. 1987, p. 429.
2. Woo, S. Injury and repair of the musculoskeletal soft tissues. Park Ridge, IL: *American Academy of Orthopaedic Surgeons. 19*87, p. 468.
3. Woo, S. Injury and repair of the musculoskeletal soft tissues. Park Ridge, IL: *American Academy of Orthopaedic Surgeons. 19*87, p. 475.
4. Woo, S. Injury and repair of the musculoskeletal soft tissues. Park Ridge, IL: *American Academy of Orthopaedic Surgeons. 19*87, p. 476.
5. Aigner, R. *Arthroscopy of the Knee.* New York, NY: Thieme Medical Publishers, Inc.. 1991, p. 74.
6. Woo, S. Injury and repair of the musculoskeletal soft tissues. Park Ridge, IL: *American Academy of Orthopaedic Surgeons. 19*87, p. 510.
7. Rowley, D. *The Musculoskeletal System.* New York, NY: Chapman & Hall Medical. 1997, p. 253.

8. Jensen, N. Arthroscopic repair of the ruptured meniscus: one to 6.3 years follow-up. *Arthroscopy.* 1994; 10:211-214.

9. Woo, S. Injury and repair of the musculoskeletal soft tissues. Park Ridge, IL: *American Academy of Orthopaedic Surgeons. 198*7, p. 517.

10. Austin, K. Complications of arthroscopic meniscal repair. *American Journal of Sports Medicine.* 1993; 21:864-868.

11. Cyriax, J. Textbook of *Orthopaedic Medicine, Volume One*: Diagnosis of Soft Tissue Lesions. Eighth Edition. Philadelphia, PA: Bailiere Tindall. 1982, p. 402.

12. Aigner, R. *Arthroscopy of the Knee.* New York, NY: Thieme Medical Publishers. 1991, p. 18.

13. Woo, S. Injury and repair of the musculoskeletal soft tissues. Park Ridge, IL: *American Academy of Orthopaedic Surgeons. 198*7, p. 513.

14. Henning, C. Arthroscopic meniscal repair using an exogenous fibrin clot. *Clinical Orthopedics.* 1990; 252:64-72.

15. Austin, K. Complications of arthroscopic meniscal repair. *American Journal of Sports Medicine.* 1993; 21:864-868.

16. Woo, S. Injury and repair of the musculoskeletal soft tissues. Park Ridge, IL: *American Academy of Orthopaedic Surgeons. 198*7, p. 512.

17. Woo, S. Injury and repair of the musculoskeletal soft tissues. Park Ridge, IL: *American Academy of Orthopaedic Surgeons. 198*7, p. 508.

18. Rubman, M. Arthroscopic repair of meniscal tears that extend into the vascular zone. A review of 198 single and complex tears. *American Journal of Sports Medicine.* 1998; 26:87-95.

19. Eggli, S. Long-term results of arthroscopic meniscal repair. An analysis of isolated tears. *American Journal of Sports Medicine.* 1995; 23:715-720.

20. Woo, S. Injury and repair of the musculoskeletal soft tissues. Park Ridge, IL: *American Academy of Orthopaedic Surgeons. 198*7, p. 522.

21. Woo, S. Injury and repair of the musculoskeletal soft tissues. Park Ridge, IL: *American Academy of Orthopaedic Surgeons. 198*7, p. 527.

22. Scott, W. *Dr. Scott's Knee Book.* New York, NY: Fireside. 1996, p. 73.

23. Rowley, D. *The Musculoskeletal System.* New York, NY: Chapman & Hall Medical. 1997, p. 246.

24. Woo, S. Injury and repair of the musculoskeletal soft tissues. Park Ridge, IL: *American Academy of Orthopaedic Surgeons. 198*7, p. 106.

25. *Clin. Orthop.* 1990; 259:192-199.

26. Scott, W. *Dr. Scott's Knee Book.* New York, NY: Fireside. 1996, p. 75.

27. Scott, W. *Dr. Scott's Knee Book.* New York, NY: Fireside. 1996, p.75.

28. Feretti, A. Osteoarthritis of the knee after ACL reconstruction. *Int. Orthop.* 1991; 15:367-371.

29. Torg, J. Natural history of the posterior cruciate ligament-deficient knee. *Clinical Orthopaedics.* 1989; 246:208-216.

30. Scott, W. *Dr. Scott's Knee Book.* New York, NY: Fireside. 1996, p. 74.

31. Lysholm, J. Long-term results after early treatment of knee injuries. *Acta Orthop Scand.* 1982; 53:109-118.

32. Tria, A. *Ligaments of the Knee.* New York, NY: Churchill Livingstone Inc., 1995, p. 167.

33. Liu, Y. An in situ study of the influence of a sclerosing solution in rabbit medial collateral ligaments and its junction strength. *Connective Tissue Research.* 1983; 2:95-102.

34. Paulos, L. The Gore-tex anterior cruciate ligament prosthesis. A long-term follow-up. *American Journal of Sports Medicine.* 1992; 20:246-252.

35. Letsch, R. Replacement of the anterior cruciate ligament by a PET prosthesis (Trevira extra-strength as a salvage procedure in chronically unstable previously operated knee joints). *Unfallchirurgie.* 1994; 20:293-301.

36. Austin, K. Complications of arthroscopic meniscal repair. *American Journal of Sports Medicine.* 1993; 21:864-868.

37. Cross, M. Acute repair of injury to the anterior cruciate ligament. A long-term follow-up. *American Journal of Sports Medicine.* 1993; 21:128-131.

38. Noyes, F. Reconstruction of the anterior ligament with human allograft. Comparison of early and later results. *Journal of Bone and Joint Surgery* (American) 1996; 78: 524-537.

39. Ongley, M. Ligament instability of the knees: a new approach to treatment. *Manual Medicine.* 1988; 3:152-154.

40. Reeves, K. Randomized prospective double-blind placebo-controlled study of dextrose Prolotherapy for knee osteoarthritis with and without ACL laxity. *Alternative Therapies* 2000; 2:68-80.

CHAPTER 6

Prolo Your Knee Pain Away!

E veryone is saddened when they see or read about an athlete who had his knee blown out. This is common in athletics because athletes are often hit from the side. *(See Figure 6-1.)* Rarely do you see an athlete really come back after knee surgery, or even arthroscopy. It is for this reason that a Prolotherapist evaluates an athlete with significant knee injuries because Prolotherapy can help regenerate stronger cruciate

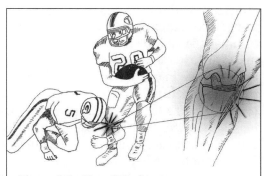

Figure 6-1: Knee Injuries
Knee injuries are common in contact sports.

ligaments, meniscal tissue, cartilage tissue, collateral ligaments, and pes anserinus tendons. Again, the referral patterns of the various ligaments around the knee should be considered. The cruciate ligaments refer pain to the back of the knee and the collateral ligaments refer pain down the leg. Though we read a lot about athletic cartilage injuries and cruciate tears, the most common condition that causes knee pain is pes anserinus tendonitis. This area, as well as the other structures of the knee, are easily treated by Prolotherapy.

PROLO GRADE 1 AND 2 LIGAMENT INJURIES AWAY!

Prolotherapy is lots of shots. It is important to know what Prolotherapy is—and what it is not. Prolotherapy is a treatment that can take partially torn ligaments and tendons and stimulate the body to repair them. What Prolotherapy is not is surgery. It cannot take a completely torn ligament and put it back together. Thus it is important for the athlete and physician to assess the severity of the ligament or tendon injury. Typically, ligament and tendon injuries are graded on a scale of 1 to 3. *(See Figure 6-2)* Grade 1 and 2 injuries still have some of the ligament fibers attached at both ends, so fibro-osseous and ligament/tendon proliferation is possible to "weld" the ends together, as Dr. Hackett put it. In grade 3 injuries, the two ends are completely separated, so surgery is often warranted in this case.

PROLOTHERAPY CAN PREVENT THE DEVELOPMENT OF TRAUMATIC ARTHRITIS

Every time an athlete collides with another athlete, or with the ground for that matter, tissue is traumatized. If a joint or ligament is traumatized and the injury does not heal, traumatic arthritis develops. Most of the old-time athletes I see in my practice have some form of traumatic arthritis. Remember that the ligaments stabilize the joints. If the ligaments are loose, then the joint is loose. The body will cause muscles to spasm to stabilize the joints. This cannot stabilize the joint; therefore the joint starts cracking. Cracking of a joint means arthritis is starting. If it periodically swells or feels painful during cold weather, arthritis is starting to form in that joint. The body will overgrow bone to stabilize the joint. This overgrowth of bone is called arthritis. *(See Figure 6-3.)* Anytime you hear the terms calcium deposit or spur, think arthritis. After thinking arthritis, when the surgeon offers to remove the spur or deposit, say "No thanks, I'll get some Prolotherapy."

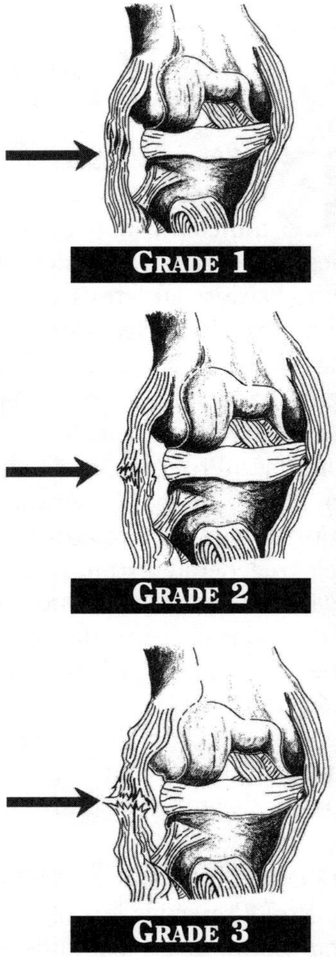

Exercise or sports do not cause arthritis; only injury to the joint causes arthritis. If aches and pains continue, the end result will be terrible traumatic arthritis. The longer treatment is delayed, the more likely an early retirement from your sport will occur. You could end up just like Bob Salerno, former Men's World Downhill Skiing Champion in the early 1970s. Ten years after the injuries, he was still not skiing because of pain. Athletes owe it

Figure 6-2: Grading of Ligament Injury Severity
Grade 1 and 2 ligament injuries are successfully treated with Prolotherapy. Grade 3 injuries, however, often need surgery.

to themselves to see the Prolotherapist rather than waiting until later when aggressive arthritis has already formed. Athletes do not have to look forward to a life ridden with the pain of arthritis, even athletes who participate in sports with very high injury rates, such as football and rugby. If injuries are given healing treatments immediately, the arthritic process can be halted. The best way to ensure this is to receive Prolotherapy.

The best time to eliminate even the remotest possibility of arthritis forming is at the time immediately following the injury. The athlete should do the now-famed **MEAT** treatments, and see a Prolotherapist for a Prolotherapy evaluation. If the ligaments are treated early with Prolotherapy, the joints strengthen and there is no longer a need for the body to grow bone spurs and calcium deposits in an attempt to stabilize loose joints and ligaments, thereby preventing the development of this type of arthritis. Prolotherapy is the only treatment I know of which can strengthen the joint and eliminate the pain of traumatic arthritis totally and completely.

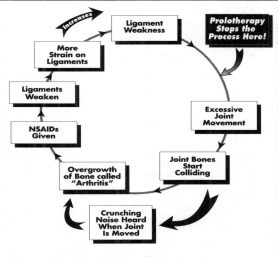

Figure 6-3: How Weakened Ligaments Lead to Arthritis
Prolotherapy stops arthritis from forming by healing the ligament weakness that started and perpetuates the cascade.

One of my patients is an avid bodybuilder, who suffered from chronically loose joints and pain. He went the route of surgery, cortisone shots, tons of anti-inflammatories, and was left with traumatic shoulder arthritis. After several treatments of Prolotherapy he told me, "My shoulder continues to become stronger and much more stable. I have no more pain, I no longer need anti-inflammatory drugs. I am able to go to the gym regularly and do exercises I could not do before, because I was frightened that my shoulder would go out and the extreme pain would come back. The Prolotherapy has ended my 15 year battle with my shoulder problems. Thanks, Doctor," he said, as he smashed me on my back. I may be a woman* of the new millennium, but why guys insist on smashing me on the back as a thank you I will never know. What happened to the good old-fashioned handshake?

PROLOTHERAPY TO CORRECT POST SURGICAL PROBLEMS AND UNSUCCESSFUL SURGERIES

Prolotherapists have bailed out many athletes and surgeons after unsuccessful surgeries. As you have already learned, surgery does not always work. I have had patients come to me after surgery who are suffering with more pain, different pain, or some remaining pain. It is amazing to me how some people succumb to multiple surgeries because each of them promised to "get at the problem." The problem with this logic is that the surgeon is depending on the MRI or CT scan to diagnose the problem. These tests measure the densities of the different tissues or the water—bone content. An athlete, above anyone else,

---

* *This chapter was written with the help of Donna Alderman, D.O., who practices Prolotherapy in California. For more information on her practice and other physicians who perform Prolotherapy, see www.getprolo.com.*

should succumb to surgery only after all other available options have been exhausted. Remember, arthroscopy is shaving, cutting, and slicing. Most surgeries involve the removal of tissue or the transferring of tissue from one area of the body to another (i.e. fusion operations or tendon transfers). Removing tissue, and moving it to another area, makes the area where the tissue was removed weaker. So in an attempt to strengthen one area, another area is weakened. Anytime you slice, cut, or dice tissue it is going to make that area of the body weaker.

Interestingly enough, when the removed tissues are sent for microscopic evaluation, they are often found to be in the *proliferating* phase. *(See Figure 6-4.)* This confirms the fact that the body's connective tissues, including cartilage, have regenerative capabilities. *(See Figure 6-5.)* It is much better for athletes to enhance their bodies' natural healing mechanisms with Prolotherapy than to remove this tissue.

If an athlete has surgery that does not resolve the pain, it means the surgery did not address the cause of the pain. Again, go back to the basics. By examining the

WEST SUBURBAN HOSPITAL MEDICAL CENTER
Erie at Austin
Oak Park, Il 60302
Phone ███████████ ███ ███████████

SURGICAL PATHOLOGY CONSULTATION REPORT

Path No. S-3826-92

Patient :   Age/Sex: 34Y F Loc. SDS
Hosp. No.: 213013   Receipt Date: 07/02/92
Physician:
History :
Procedure: Arthroscopy, Right Knee

Specimen : TISSUE, KNEE

FINAL DIAGNOSIS

TISSUE, RIGHT KNEE, ARTHROSCOPY:

FRAGMENTS OF PROLIFERATING SYNOVIAL TISSUE, FRAGMENTS OF DEGENERATING HYALINE AND FIBROCARTILAGE AND ASSOCIATED DENSE FIBROCONNECTIVE AND ADIPOSE TISSUE.

CROSS EXAMINATION

The specimen is received in formalin in a suction bag labeled "tissue, right knee" and consists of fragments of cartilaginous tissue admixed with fragments of adipose tissue. The specimen aggregates to 2 x 2 x 0.8 cm. Representative sections are placed in a single cassette.
pz/ecp

PATHOLOGIST

Date reported July 6, 1992

SURGICAL PATHOLOGY REPORT (page 1)

Figure 6-4: Arthroscopic Tissue Analysis
Notice that the microscopic tissue analysis revealed proliferating tissue. This indicates that a repair process was stopped by removal of the tissue. A better approach is stimulating the connective tissue to repair with Prolotherapy.

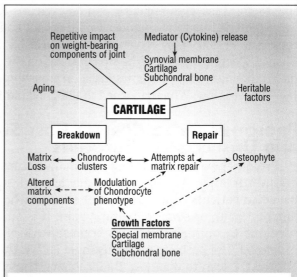

Figure 6-5: The Cartilage Repair Process
The connective tissues of the body all have regenerative properties—including the cartilage.

painful area and locating its exact location and treating it with Prolotherapy, the chronic pain, even after surgery can be totally and permanently eliminated. Prolotherapy is the only technique I know of which can potentially correct the damage caused by surgery. This is possible because by Prolotherapy injections, the ligaments around the operative site are strengthened, helping to restore normal function and decrease pain. Obviously, getting Prolotherapy instead of surgery is a better option. Prolotherapy cannot always totally repair a surgerized area, but it can sure make it stronger. Many athletes have been surgerized and left with chronic pain only to return to athletics because of Prolotherapy.

PROLOTHERAPY CAN MAKE YOUR BODY STRONGER THAN PRIOR TO INJURY

Your body is like a fine-tuned automobile. When it breaks down, do you take it to the local chop shop or to the best mechanic you can afford? You do whatever it takes to repair the broken part in your car. A double-blinded study done at the University of Iowa used normal rabbit knee ligaments and showed that repeated injections of Prolotherapy significantly increased the mass of the ligaments by 44 percent above normal, the thickness by 27 percent, and the ligament-bone junction strength by 28 percent.[1] *(See Figure 6-6.)* A similar study done on rabbit tendons obtained similar results in only six weeks.[2] Imagine what it would mean to an athlete to run 40 percent faster, jump 40 percent higher, or be 40 percent stronger? Many athletes are finding out by getting Prolotherapy.

THE EFFECTS OF SIX PROLOTHERAPY TREATMENTS TO THE MEDIAL COLLATERAL LIGAMENT

	Prolotherapy-Injected Ligaments	Saline-Injected Ligaments (Control)	% Change
Ligament Mass (mg)	132.2	89.7	44
Ligament Thickness (mm)	1.01	0.79	27
Ligament Mass Length (mg/mm)	6.45	4.39	47
Junction Strength (N)	119.1	93.5	28

Figure 6-6: The Effects of Six Prolotherapy Treatments to the Medial Collateral Ligament
Prolotherapy causes a statistically significant increase in ligament mass and strength as well as bone-ligament junction strength.

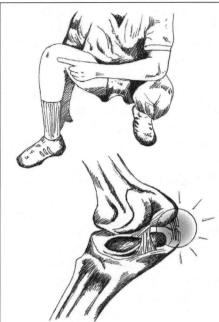

Figure 6-7: The "Positive Point Sign"
Here the athlete illustrates the exact site of the pain. This combined with the doctor's "positive jump sign" are two good indicators that Prolotherapy at that *exact* site will cure the athlete's injury.

THE KNEE DIAGNOSIS: IT IS ONLY A POKE AWAY!

How do we go about diagnosing knee problems? First, we need a good history and a thorough physical exam. There are many fancy orthopedic medicine testing maneuvers that can help locate the structure that is injured, but none is as significant as asking the patient to locate the painful area and then poking on the area to reproduce the pain. *(See Figure 6-7.)* This can diagnose most knee injuries.[3] If the history and physical examination does not reveal the source of the problem then we might consider taking pictures of the knee. There are several ways to take pictures of the knee. Plain x-rays show only the bones, how they align, how far apart they are, and if they are broken. Standing plain x-rays of the knee are generally only useful to access the amount of cartilage deterioration or growth after Prolotherapy for people with chronic pain. MRIs of the knee are becoming more common. They can show soft tissues like ligaments and meniscus. They cost about $1,400 and have an accuracy of close to 90 percent for most knee structures but should not replace a good medical history and physical exam.[4] A weakness of MRI is that it cannot see the articular cartilage. You must always remember that an MRI can never tell you what is causing the pain! Only a physician, and preferably an orthopedic medicine specialist, can tell you this!

HEALING THE KNEE: KEEPING THE FIBRO-OSSEOUS JUNCTION STRONG

There are some general principles about healing knee injuries without surgery. One of the first principles is to keep the area moving, while at the same time protecting the joint from strong stresses. Immobilization of the injured joint causes the repaired area to become weaker and thinner.[5] Immobilization of the knee often leads to a stiff joint. This is due to a combination of adhesions in the joint and/or shortening of ligaments, and weakening the site where ligaments and tendons insert to bone. This is why the **R.I.C.E.** (**R**est, **I**ce, **C**ompression, and **E**levation) treatment protocols for soft tissue injuries are so detrimental to healing. Ligaments are especially sensitive to immobility, therefore it is not recommended for any type of ligament tear or sprain when the joint itself is stable.

Interestingly, it has been shown that the more we exercise a specific joint, the stronger the bone-ligament and bone-tendon complexes become![6] Exercise specifically helps strengthen the fibro-osseous junction, which is where the ligament/tendon and bone attach to each other. Controlled activity is therefore an important part of preventing injury and healing from injury! In one study on animals, the investigators found that trained animals had ligaments with thickened collagen fiber bundles, more collagen, and increased strength than their non-trained animal colleagues.[7] It is at and immediately around this critical junction, the ligament-bone junction, that most injuries occur.[8] This is another reason why Prolotherapy is so effective at curing sports injuries and enhancing athletic performance because it stimulates the body to repair the ligaments and tendons at the fibro-osseous junction, exactly where the weakness is located.

It turns out that there are other substances that promote healing of knee injuries, such as hormones. Some of these are Growth Hormone, thyroid hormone, testosterone, dehydroepiandrosterone (DHEA), and others. When one or more of these hormones are deficient, healing is delayed.[9] When deficient hormones are replaced, the body has a much greater capacity to heal. If indicated, doctors who practice natural medicine will often test the person in pain for these deficiencies and replace them as necessary. Hormone testing is generally indicated for anyone over the age of 45. It is my opinion that natural hormone replacement should be done in women and men. Men around the country, especially the athletic ones, are finding out just how young and athletic they can be while taking natural testosterone and other hormones. These hormones help sustain vitality in both sexes, as well as enhance sports performance. For younger athletes there are nutritional products and secretagogues that can help enhance secretion of the hormones. For this reason many athletes are seeing physicians who practice natural medicine along with Prolotherapy.

Even though adequate hormones, proper nutrition, and exercise are of vital importance for healing sports injuries, there is nothing more powerful to heal sports injuries than Prolotherapy. Prolotherapy involves the injection of substances at the fibro-osseous junctions of ligaments and tendons to induce the

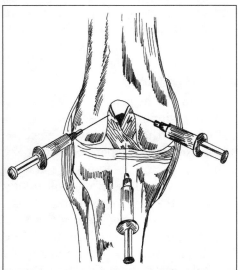

Figure 6-8: Prolotherapy of the Knee
Prolotherapy is effective for injuries to the knee ligaments, tendons, menisci, and cartilage.

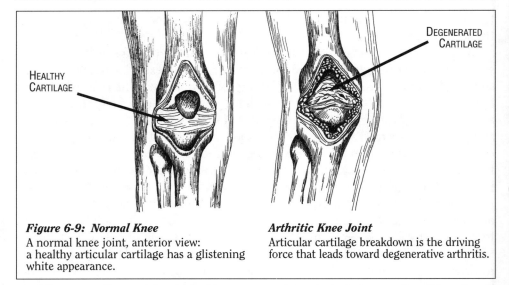

Figure 6-9: Normal Knee
A normal knee joint, anterior view:
a healthy articular cartilage has a glistening
white appearance.

Arthritic Knee Joint
Articular cartilage breakdown is the driving
force that leads toward degenerative arthritis.

proliferation of normal strong ligament and tendon tissue at the exact site of the injection. *(See Figure 6-8.)* This makes joints, like the knee, stronger. Once the knee joint is strong, the athlete has no more pain, as well as enhanced athletic performance. With this in mind, I will now describe various injuries to the knee and show how Prolotherapy can help the athlete be more active and have complete pain relief. I believe, after reading this chapter, you will say it is true, "You can Prolo your knee injuries away!"

The number one cause of knee pain that I see is degenerative arthritis. The reason, as you may have guessed, as to why so many people have degenerative knee arthritis is because they took years of NSAIDs and cortisone shots which deteriorated their menisci and cartilage.

DEGENERATIVE JOINT DISEASE VERSUS AGING

Getting old has nothing to do with getting pain! Many people come in to the office, doubtful that anything could help them, resigning themselves to living with chronic pain because they are older. Hogwash! There is always a cause for chronic pain. The cause is not old age. This is exemplified when looking at the articular cartilage in the joints of an older person versus the joints of someone with osteoarthritis (degenerative arthritis) at any age. The joints look totally and completely different! The articular cartilage of the aging person looks nothing like the articular cartilage of a patient with arthritis. *(See Figure 6-9.)*

Pain is the body's signal that something is wrong, weakened, or injured. The most commonly injured tissues in the chronic pain sufferer are the ligaments that stabilize the joints. It is the laxity or weakness in these tissues that produces most degenerative joint disease.

The bones in a joint such as the knee are no longer held in a stable position following an injury to the ligaments. This leads to instability in the knee with

82

PROLOTHERAPY VERSUS SURGERY

What would you rather have done to relieve your pain? Surgery or Prolotherapy?

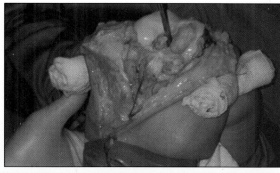

A Total Knee Replacement

A picture of back surgery in process.

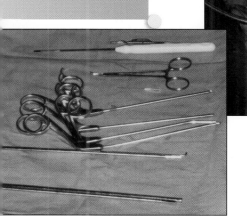

The Assault—Tools of Surgery

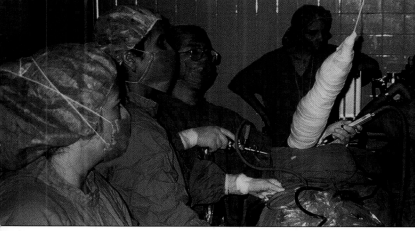

Arthroscopy of the Shoulder: Notice that it takes five people to perform this "safe" procedure...

PROLOTHERAPY VERSUS ARTHROSCOPY

Prolotherapy versus Arthroscopy Chart

	PROLOTHERAPY	ARTHROSCOPY
Stimulates repair?	Yes	No
Increases collagen strength?	Yes	No
Arthritis risk?	Decreased	Increased
Return to sport?	Quick	Slow
Rehabilitation time?	Short	Long
Exercise?	Encouraged	Cautious
Anesthesia required?	No	Yes
Cost?	Hundreds	Thousands
Time involved in procedure?	Minutes	Hours
Instruments used?	Thin needles	Massive Scopes

Prolotherapy has many advantages over arthroscopy; so why are so many people with knee pain receiving arthroscopies?

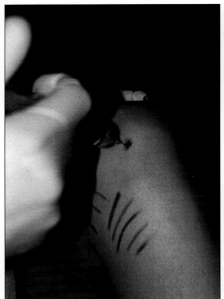

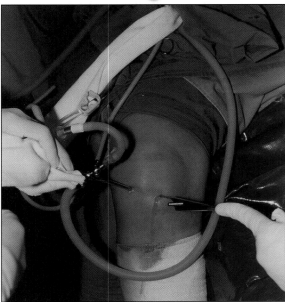

Prolotherapy on the Knee
Prolotherapy of the Knee involves one needle and lots of smiles.

Arthroscopy: Notice all the tubes and instruments needed for knee arthroscopy...

Every surgery or arthroscopy begins with the knife...

PROLOTHERAPY STIMULATES CARTILAGE AND MENISCI REPAIR

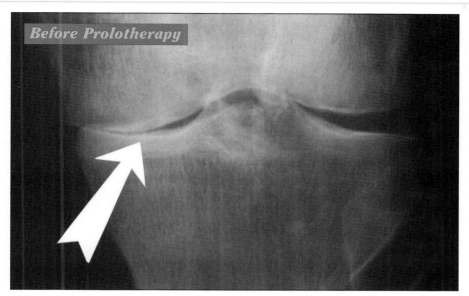

Before Prolotherapy, this x-ray shows advanced degenerative arthritis—the so-called bone-on-bone phenomenon.

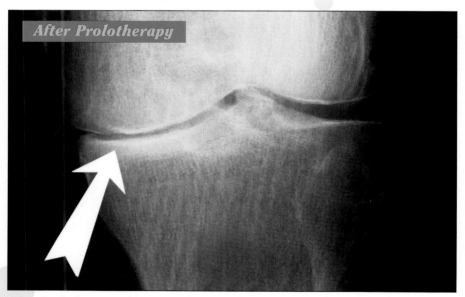

After Prolotherapy: this x-ray shows evidence of cartilage repair. The joint is no longer bone-on-bone.

The above x-rays were taken before and after 12 Prolotherapy sessions. The person went from limping and walking with a cane to *unlimited* mobility because of Prolotherapy.

PROLOTHERAPY: THE SCIENCE

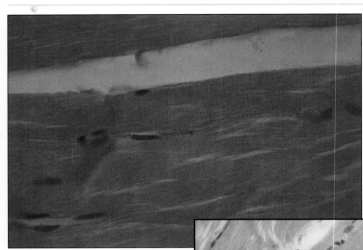

On the left:
Normal Muscle Tissue
(Prior to Prolotherapy)

Below: Muscle tissue
96 hours after an injection
with 12.5% dextrose and
0.5% xylocaine.

Note the high concentration
of fibroblasts, indicative
of a good inflammatory
reaction. This is the
basic Hackett-Hemwall
Prolotherapy solution.

Below left: Muscle tissue
96 hours after an injection
with 12.5% dextrose and an
equal amount of 1%
xylocaine, 2.5% phenol, and
12.5% glycerine. The
inflammatory reaction is
substantial in comparison with
the middle photo. This is the
Prolotherapy solution
known as P2G.

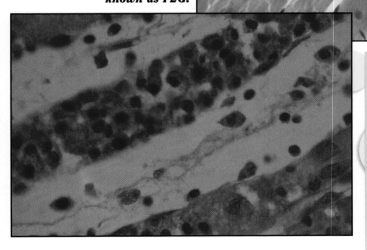

Prolotherapy stimulates the body to repair the painful areas. The various solutions when injected into the injured areas, induce the normal inflammatory cascade to help heal such tissues as ligaments, tendons, discs, and cartilage.

Photos compliments of K. Dean Reeves, M.D. Slides made by Gale Bordon, M.D., and given to various members of the Prolotherapy Association in the 1960's. Dr. Bordon's research into the histology of Prolotherapy was presented at the annual Clinical Symposium of the Prolotherapy Association, June 16, 1968, Bellevue Hotel, San Francisco, California. Used with permission from Yvonne Bordon.

eventual crunching in the joint. Crunching in a joint is a sure sign that the joint-stabilizing structures are in a weakened state. A person who receives Prolotherapy at this point can stop this whole downward spiral. If the joint instability is not treated, the degeneration in the joint will continue. Eventually this will lead to articular cartilage breakdown. Even at this point, Prolotherapy, in conjunction with nutritional remedies can help regenerate the injured tissue. If left untreated, all of the articular cartilage will erode and the person will be left with a joint that is stiff and painful. The orthopedist will call the condition "bone on bone." Prolotherapy can still be tried for "bone on bone" but it is not as successful as when the degenerative process is only mild to moderate. These patients typically experience some pain relief, but not complete relief. To some people, partial pain relief is worth it.

Degenerative joint conditions almost always start because of a soft tissue injury to the joint. Generally this is an injury to the ligaments, the stabilizing structures of the joint. When the ligaments are stretched and weakened, the other structures in the joint must perform functions that they were not designed to do. Eventually these structures become fatigued and cartilage begins to break down. This process is commonly experienced in the hip and knee joints. This is the reason why over 120,000 hip replacements and 95,000 knee replacements are performed each year in the United States alone.[10, 11]

CAUSES OF OSTEOARTHRITIS

Osteoarthritis almost always begins as ligament weakness. *(See Figure 6-10.)* Joints are composed of two bones covered with articular cartilage, allowing the joint to glide, and ligaments holding the two bones together. Healthy articular cartilage and ligaments enable the two bones to glide evenly over one another when the bones move.

If the ligaments become weak, the bones will glide over one another in an uneven manner. One area of the bone will bear additional weight on the articular cartilage when the joint is stressed. This uneven distribution of joint stress creates an even greater strain on the weakened ligament in order to stabilize this joint. Eventually all of the ligaments of the joint become lax. The more lax the ligaments become, the more unstable the joint. This increases the abnormal weight distribution inside the joint. This continued stress within the joint causes articular cartilage breakdown which causes the bones to glide roughly over each other producing a crunching noise when the joint is moved. Grinding or crunching is a warning sign that a cortisone shot awaits you at your conventional doctor's office, unless something is done.

At some point in this process, the body realizes the ligaments can no longer stabilize the joint. Muscles and their respective tendons will then tense in an attempt to stabilize the area on the weakened side of the joint, adding to the person's discomfort. As the muscles and their tendons weaken, which will occur over time, they become more painful and unable to stabilize the joint. They will often

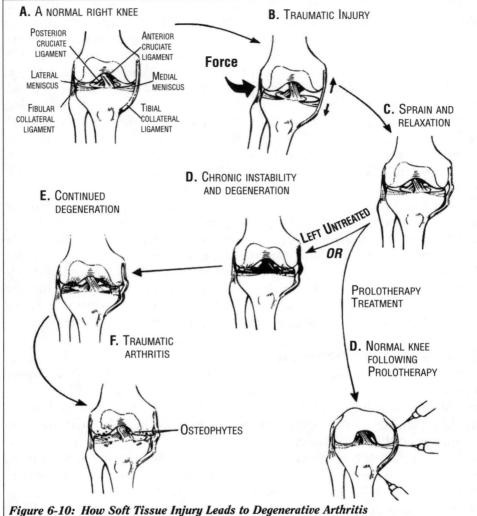

A. A NORMAL RIGHT KNEE

POSTERIOR CRUCIATE LIGAMENT

ANTERIOR CRUCIATE LIGAMENT

LATERAL MENISCUS

MEDIAL MENISCUS

FIBULAR COLLATERAL LIGAMENT

TIBIAL COLLATERAL LIGAMENT

B. TRAUMATIC INJURY

Force

C. SPRAIN AND RELAXATION

D. CHRONIC INSTABILITY AND DEGENERATION

E. CONTINUED DEGENERATION

LEFT UNTREATED

OR

PROLOTHERAPY TREATMENT

F. TRAUMATIC ARTHRITIS

D. NORMAL KNEE FOLLOWING PROLOTHERAPY

OSTEOPHYTES

Figure 6-10: How Soft Tissue Injury Leads to Degenerative Arthritis
Following trauma, ligaments become sprained. When healing does not occur, the ligaments become relaxed, resulting in chronic instability and degeneration. When left untreated, post-traumatic "arthritis," or degeneration follows. This degenerative process can be prevented with appropriate intervention through Prolotherapy.

"knot" producing painful trigger points. When the muscles and ligaments can no longer stabilize the joint, the bony surfaces rub against each other as the menisci and cartilage deteriorate. In a last attempt to stabilize the joint, additional bone begins accumulating where the bones collide. This bony overgrowth is called osteoarthritis. Eventually, if the process is not stopped at some point, a stiff joint will form. *(See Figure 6-11.)*

At any time during this process, the body can quickly stabilize the joint by swelling. Swelling of a joint indicates the presence of some foreign substance

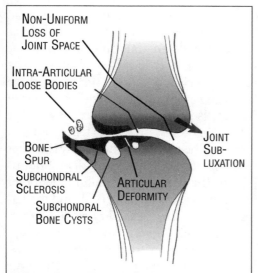

NON-UNIFORM
LOSS OF
JOINT SPACE

INTRA-ARTICULAR
LOOSE BODIES

BONE
SPUR

SUBCHONDRAL
SCLEROSIS

SUBCHONDRAL
BONE CYSTS

ARTICULAR
DEFORMITY

JOINT
SUB-
LUXATION

Figure 6-11: Knee Arthritis
Knee arthritis is generally characterized by
a loss of joint space because of meniscal and
articular cartilage degeneration. It is this
degeneration and the bone spurs that cause
the knee joint to feel stiff.

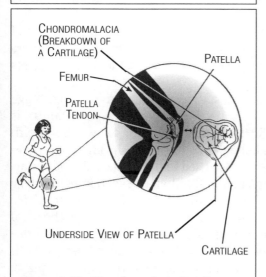

CHONDROMALACIA
(BREAKDOWN OF
A CARTILAGE)

FEMUR

PATELLA
TENDON

PATELLA

UNDERSIDE VIEW OF PATELLA

CARTILAGE

Figure 6-12: Chondromalacia Patella
This condition involves cartilage deterioration
beneath the patella.

**Used with permission by G. Gaten, from Play Healthy,
Stay Healthy, Human Kinetics, 1991.**

inside the joint or that the joint is
loose. Microorganisms, such as bac-
teria, blood, pieces of cartilage, and
various bodily breakdown products
can accumulate in the joints and
cause swelling. If a tissue is injured
inside and around the joint, typically the joint swells as a protective
measure so the body can repair the
tissue, which may eventually lead
to the development of arthritis.
Swelling of a joint typically means
that a structure inside the joint has
been injured. The best treatment to
repair structures in the knee joint,
including the menisci and articular
cartilage is Prolotherapy.

PATELLOFEMORAL PAIN SYNDROME

Anterior knee pain is the most
common presenting symptom from
an athlete in a clinical sports medicine practice.[12] Patellofemoral pain
syndrome (PFPS) is the term used to
describe a continuum of articular
cartilage changes affecting the
underside of the patella. The condition is sometimes referred to as
chondromalacia patella. "Chondro"
means cartilage, "malacia" means
degeneration, and "patella" is the
patella, or kneecap. Chrondromal-
acia patella (also known as PFPS) is
therefore a condition whereby cartilage damage beneath the patella
(kneecap) occurs. *(See Figure
6-12.)* The primary symptom in
PFPS is anterior knee pain. It is possible to have PFPS with no cartilage
damage in the knee. In this instance,
many would call the condition
"patello-femoral tracking syndrome"

85

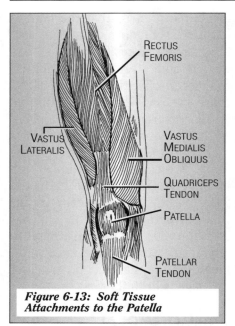

RECTUS
FEMORIS

VASTUS
LATERALIS

VASTUS
MEDIALIS
OBLIQUUS

QUADRICEPS
TENDON

PATELLA

PATELLAR
TENDON

***Figure 6-13: Soft Tissue
Attachments to the Patella***

because the problem is due to abnormal tracking of the patella.

The patellofemoral joints act as pulley systems for the lower extremities. The patella consists of a bony surface of three facets and a central ridge. The underside of the patella should be in alignment with the femoral groove. The soft tissue attachments of the patella include the quadriceps tendons, the vastus medialis obliquus (VMO), the medial retinaculum, adductor fibers, the vastus lateralis (VL), and the lateral retinaculum.[13] ***(See Figure 6-13.)***

The patellofemoral joint absorbs significant forces with different activities. While walking on a level surface the force is one-half the body weight. Climbing stairs exerts a force three to four times the body weight. Squatting puts a force through the knee joint at seven to eight times the body weight. Imagine the force through the patellofemoral joint during a wrestling takedown or lifting 300 pounds during a squat lift.[12]

Patellofemoral contact occurs during various stages of knee flexion. At full extension, the patella and femur have no contact. The greatest contact occurs at 90 degrees of flexion in the superior position. The medial and lateral facets make no contact until 135 degrees.

PFPS generally causes no other symptoms, except pain, until some cartilage damage on the underside of the patella occurs. A grinding noise, or crepitus, is heard in the knee when this occurs. Ross has this condition. He was born with a crooked right foot because the tibia bone points outward. His kneecap, therefore, does not correctly track on the femur. He used to have knee pain, but treated the condition with nutritional supplements that helped regenerate cartilage and received Prolotherapy from Drs. Rodney Van Pelt and Mark Wheaton.* He has no pain whatsoever at this point in time, except when we go into withdrawal and order an Edwardo's famous spinach-stuffed Chicago-style pizza. The knee pain will then mysteriously appear. The reason for this is because Ross has both a wheat and a dairy allergy, both of which are contained in Edwardo's pizza. Interestingly enough, some people have pain in only one joint due to food allergy. This is why we sometimes test athletes for food allergies when they come to our office with sports injuries.

---

* *Dr. Van Pelt practices Prolotherapy in California and Dr. Wheaton in Minnesota. For more information, please see www.getprolo.com.*

TREATMENT OF PFPS

Traditional sports medicine treats PFPS with the following: taping, medial quadriceps muscle exercises, electrical stimulation, massage, bracing, interferential treatments, cortisone shots, orthotics, NSAIDs, exercise, and a host of other treatments. The whole theory of the condition is based on the fact that one of the following musculoskeletal abnormalities exists and if it is corrected, the athlete will feel much better: patella alta/baja, tibial external rotation, tight hamstrings, poor VMO/VL timing, femoral anteversion, subtalar pronation, narrow femoral trochlea/groove, genu varus/valgus, tight iliotibial band, poor patellar mobility, or some kind of an adhesion.[13]

Dr. Bruce Arroll and associates produced a high-quality evidence-based review of successful treatments based on outcome information, because so many therapies were advocated for treating PFPS.[14] They reviewed more than 50 articles on this condition and found only five papers which met the inclusion criteria of being randomized controlled trials.

One of the studies by Finestone examined 395 male infantry recruits during basic training. Fifty-nine of the recruits developed PFPS. The intervention group was given an elastic knee sleeve with a silicone patellar ring, presumably to hold it in place so it tracks better. The other group was given a simple elastic knee sleeve to wear. The no-treatment group wore no sleeve. The no-treatment group had the lowest mean pain score at the end of the study and was statistically significantly lower than either of the two groups wearing the elastic sleeves.[15] The study also revealed that 18 percent of the knees in the simple sleeve group and 55 percent of the knees in the elastic knee sleeve with a silicone patellar ring developed discomfort or local skin abrasions secondary to wearing the braces. Dr. Bruce Arroll wrote in his journal article that **"knee braces and sleeves should be avoided"** for PFPS.[14]

Kannus and associates divided their study group into three different groups: an intervention group receiving intra-articular glycosaminoglycan polysulfate; a control group receiving intra-articular physiologic saline; and a non-injection group. Both injection groups were given local anesthesia with lidocaine combined with the glycosaminoglycan polysulfate or saline. At the six-week assessment, the two injection groups were **significantly better** than the non-injection group on all three patellar assessments and full-squatting tests. At six months, the amount of pain experienced was significantly less in the injection groups.[16] Remember that glycosaminoglycans are the components of cartilage that attract water and give the compressive and load-bearing effects to the cartilage. With only one injection, people with PFPS received significant pain relief.

Why did this occur? This occurred because there was a deficiency in the cartilage of the PFPS patients. None of the other treatments, such as exercise, NSAIDs, cortisone shots, taping, bracing, etc., do anything to help rebuild the cartilage. Patellofemoral pain syndrome or chondromalacia patella must be viewed as a localized connective tissue deficiency of the cartilage. This is why people with this condition, or any cartilage deterioration, who come to our office usually receive Prolotherapy with glucosamine added to the solution. Glucosamine is one of the components of the glycosaminoglycans. The only difference between our treatment and the above study is that the person with PFPS receives the glucosamine directly into the joint with each treatment on multiple visits.

Raatikainen and associates had a similar idea, but gave glycosaminoglycan polysulfate intramuscularly. Patients with retropatellar cartilage damage (chondromalacia patella) were studied for 12 months. The glycosaminoglycan polysulfate injection caused statistically significant improvements, as seen on the surfaces of the cartilage at the 12-month arthroscopic evaluation.[17] This would be expected because this type of approach gets at the root cause of the problem, which is cartilage deterioration. The cartilage needs certain substrates in order to regenerate and one of them is glycosaminoglycan.

People with PFPS often experience a myriad of musculoskeletal abnormalities around the knee. This includes an increased Q-angle and weakness in the vastus medialis and tightness in the lateral retinaculum. Many athletic trainers and physiotherapists get what they consider to be great results by using tailored exercise with taping and bracing programs. The patients who come to my office have obviously tried these methods with limited success. Many people receive some help, but few are cured by the traditional sports medicine approach to this condition.

I was cured of my PFPS pain with Prolotherapy to the point where I broke four hours in the Milwaukee Marathon—despite limping in pain five months before the race due to a flare-up of the chondromalacia patella and an ACL tear. The remarkable healing that occurs with conditions like these can only occur with Prolotherapy. Prolotherapy injections are given at the direct site of the problem—inside the joint where the cartilage is deteriorating. Prolotherapy presumably works by stimulating the proliferation of chondrocytes, causing a change in their status to chondroblastic cells which are more capable of undergoing proliferation, or growth. The main effect for the athlete is a dramatic improvement in the pain levels. Treatments are continued until complete pain relief is obtained, usually necessitating four to eight sessions. Because the condition involves cartilage degeneration, glucosamine may be added to the standard proliferant solution. Nutritional supplements such as cod liver oil, bromelain, MSM, glucosamine, chondroitin sulfate, and/or ProloMax may also be given.* Prolotherapy in conjunction with appropriate nutritional supplementation can cure chronic knee pain that wrestlers and other athletes commonly experience. This offers hope for many athletes who have given up on ever competing again.

---

* For a complete list of the supplements I reccommend to assist soft tissue healing, see **Appendix G**.

THE OVERUSE SYNDROME THEORY: THE TRADITIONAL MODEL

Traditional sports medicine believes that the majority of sports injuries occur by overuse.[18] For this reason, various treatment modalities such as cessation of activities, the **RICE** protocol, and NSAIDs are prescribed.

It is easy to understand this point of view when the amount of force athletes put on their bodies is analyzed. Consider the fact that the foot touches the soil between 800 to 2,000 times on a one-mile run. The ground reactive force at midstance in running is 250 to 300 percent of body weight. A 70-kilogram (150 pound) runner at 1,175 steps per mile absorbs at least 220 tons of force per mile.[19] The overuse theory seems to make sense because even the smallest anatomical or biomechanical abnormalities of the lower extremities, especially if they are subjected to training errors or some other external factors, could lead to overuse injuries of the lower extremities and/or the spine.

To understand the genesis of overuse injuries in the upper extremities, one should only ponder, for a couple of seconds, the number of times a javelin thrower throws his spear, a weight lifter lifts his weights, or a handball or water polo player takes a shot at the goal. To cite an example, a swimmer will typically make somewhere in the neighborhood of 4,000 overhead strokes during one training session. This adds up to more than 800,000 overhead strokes in just one season and simply illustrates why around 60 percent of the top-class swimmers suffer from overuse injury in the shoulder area.[20]

An overuse injury is said to occur when a repetitive microtrauma overloads the capacity of a tissue to repair itself. This results in an inflammatory response leading to acute, and then possibly chronic, inflammation resulting in structural changes in the tissues. The inflammation is usually associated with swelling, redness, increased temperature, and tenderness. These signs may be present if superficial structures are inflamed. Inflammation of deeper structures, however, may not necessarily demonstrate these signs.[21] This is definitely true! When examined, the athletes often do not exhibit signs of inflammation. There is no redness, no swelling, no increased temperature, but yes, oh yes, they have tenderness upon palpation.

The main problem with the traditional overuse syndrome theory is that the treatment of **RICE** and NSAIDs does reduce pain for a time, but the condition eventually returns. This is why you have so many athletes with chronic nagging injuries. Many of them are prematurely ending their careers. The problem with the overuse syndrome theory is that it is wrong! There is a much better approach which gives much longer-lasting results.

CONNECTIVE TISSUE DEFICIENCY SYNDROME (CTDS): A NATURAL MEDICINE VIEW

Exercise that elicits the most soreness is generally comprised of unaccustomed eccentric muscle contractions. Eccentric contractions are those in which the muscle lengthens as it creates tension. This is what occurs in the

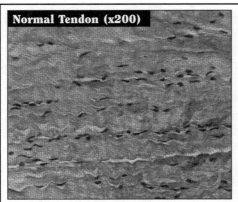 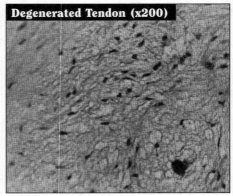

Figure 6-14: Comparison of Normal and Degenerated Tendon
The slide on the right is indicative of chronic Achilles and patellar tendon injuries. The injuries are often called tendonitis, but a better term is tendinosis, because the overwhelming histology is degeneration—not inflammation.

Used by permission of Mark Pecina & Ivan Bojanic, CRC Press ©1993 Boca Raton, FL. Overuse injuries of the musculoskeletal system.

quadriceps muscle as a runner runs downhill. An eccentric action occurs during a biceps curl exercise when the lifter lowers the weight as the arm extends.

What exactly causes the muscle soreness after exercise? Is it a muscle spasm, a muscle tear, or degeneration? It turns out that when muscle biopsies are taken from subjects who experience sore muscles, there is definite evidence of muscle fiber disruption and degeneration.[22-25] It is this degeneration or disruption that stimulates the regrowth or regeneration of the muscle, which produces a stronger and bigger muscle. It is also evident that muscles are breaking down with exercise because the common blood markers of muscle damage—creatine kinase, myoglobin, and lactate dehydrogenase—increase manifold during exercise.[26-28]

This same degeneration is found with tendons. When examined under the microscope, the athletes' injured tendons look degenerated from long-term exercise, they were not inflamed.[29-31] There is evidence of scarring and a random organization of collagen fibers. *(See Figure 6-14.)* Parts of the tendon become acellular. An interesting point is that there is one type of tissue that does appear to become inflamed and that is the nervous tissue in the area of the injured tendon or in the area of its insertion. Following tendon injury, the presence of perineuritis is accompanied by an increase in the breadth of the nerve sheath which laterally compresses the nerve.[32] This may explain why Neural Therapy, in conjunction with Prolotherapy, is so effective at stimulating healing after sports injuries. This also explains why some Prolotherapists put Sarapin, an extract of the pitcher plant, into their solutions. This particular natural substance is extremely effective at helping calm nerve pain and enhance healing of neuritis (inflammation of the nerve).

Sports injuries that linger more than a couple of weeks should be examined from a connective tissue standpoint. Ligaments, tendons, and muscles are made up of cells called fibroblasts, which produce the collagen and ground substance

FIGURE 6-15: FACTORS AFFECTING HEALING OF CONNECTIVE TISSUE

- AGE
- GENDER
- TYPE OF INJURY
- SEVERITY OF INJURY
- UNDERLYING DISEASE PROCESSES
- HORMONAL INFLUENCES
- DIETARY INTAKE
- NUTRITIONAL STATUS
- DEGREE OF HYPOXIA (SYSTEMIC AND LOCAL)

- TYPE OF TISSUE(S) AFFECTED
- ELECTRICAL FIELDS
- MECHANICAL LOAD FORCES
- TEMPERATURE
- PHARMACOLOGICAL AGENTS (DRUGS)
- MOBILITY (LOCAL AND WHOLE-BODY)
- TYPE OF ONSET (ACUTE OR CHRONIC)

- STRUCTURAL (PHYSICAL) DEFORMITIES
- PHYSIOLOGICAL INFLUENCES (PLACEBO EFFECTS AND PSYCHO-NEURO-IMMUNOLOGICAL LINKS)
- METABOLIC AND CELL TURNOVER RATES OF CONNECTIVE TISSUES
- MUSCULAR STRENGTHS AND FORCES
- BLOOD SUPPLY

- OVERALL HEALTH STATUS
- TIMING OF RETURN TO PHYSICAL ACTIVITY
- pH AND LACTATE CONCENTRATION
- GROWTH FACTORS, CYTOKINES, EICOSANOIDS

Adapted from **Nutrition Applied to Injury Rehabilitation and Sports Medicine** *by L. Bucci, CRC Press, Boca Raton, FL ©1995.*

(proteoglycans) that make up the tissues. With chronic sports injury, a deficiency in the amount of collagen and proteoglycans that are being made by the fibroblasts is seen for some reason. If the fibroblasts are stimulated to make more collagen and proteoglycans, the injured tissue will subsequently be rebuilt. The end result will be a stronger, thicker ligament or tendon. This will make the athletes stronger and their athletic performance will be enhanced. There are various causes as to why the fibroblasts do not generate enough collagen and proteoglycans. This is shown in *Figure 6-15.*

The sports medicine physician is responsible for determining which of the above factors might be missing in the athlete with the non-healing injury. At Caring Medical and Rehabilitation Services in Oak Park, Illinois, the athlete is put through a nutritional testing protocol called Metabolic Typing to determine the specific individual nutritional and dietary needs. It is important to remember that there is no one diet that is best for every person. Each person should be treated individually. Other testing may include hormonal testing, comprehensive stool analysis looking for intestinal dysbiosis and nutrient absorption problems (ensuring that the gastrointestinal tract is healthy, allowing proper digestion and absorption), and other testing as needed to provide the athlete with the maximum ability to heal. This is the future of sports medicine. It is no longer about suppressing the symptoms with NSAIDs. It is the sports medicine physician's job to allow the athlete to heal the sports injury by correcting connective tissue deficiency. This makes a lot more sense than "covering up" the symptoms of the deficiency by giving NSAIDs.

Tendinosis or tendon degeneration and ligament laxities go hand in hand. They can make each other worse or be the etiological basis for the other. When a tendon is injured or degenerated, the ligament no longer has dynamic support in the joint. Likewise, if a ligament is degenerated or lax, the joint becomes unstable, meaning that the tendon has no static support. It must now be the static and dynamic stabilizer. Eventually it degenerates. *(See Figure 6-16.)*

Prolotherapy is administered directly to the injured areas, which stimulates the fibroblasts that make the new connective tissue. *Both* the ligaments and tendons get stronger. Many athletes who have been told they have "chronic tendonitis" actually have tendinosis or degenerated tendon. When biopsies are taken of areas that have been chronically painful and injured they do not show inflammation but degeneration.

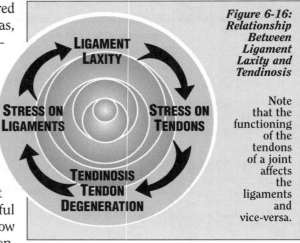

Figure 6-16: Relationship Between Ligament Laxity and Tendinosis

Note that the functioning of the tendons of a joint affects the ligaments and vice-versa.

The important point to make is that injured tissues needs to be stimulated to repair itself. What the person needs to heal the area is some inflammatory cells in their to lay down some new collagen. Prolotherapy is the best treatment to stimulate the fibroblasts, which initiate collagen proliferation. The tendinosis is turned into a tendonitis (on purpose) and eventually a strong tendon is made. *(See Figure 6-17.)* This is why the treatment is called Prolotherapy, because it proliferates fibroblasts, which proliferate collagen and proteoglycans, which proliferate ligaments and tendons, making them stronger and thicker. Once the athletes' ligaments and tendons are thicker and stronger, not only do they not have to decrease their hours of training or reduce their miles of running, they can actually increase them! Do you see the difference between the old theory and the new theory? *(See Figure 6-18.)*

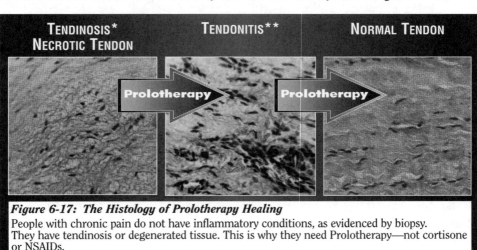

Figure 6-17: The Histology of Prolotherapy Healing
People with chronic pain do not have inflammatory conditions, as evidenced by biopsy.
They have tendinosis or degenerated tissue. This is why they need Prolotherapy—not cortisone or NSAIDs.

Used with permission from Overuse Injuries of the Musculoskeletal System—*Marko M. Peling, CRC Press, 1993, Boca Raton, FL.*
 *Biopsy of tendon of athlete with "overuse injury."
**Biopsy of tendon showing tendonitis. This is what occurs immediately after Prolotherapy.

FIGURE 6-18: CONNECTIVE TISSUE DEFICIENCY SYNDROME (CTDS) VERSUS OVERUSE SYNDROME

	CTDS (NEW VIEW)	OVERUSE (OLD VIEW)
Cause of the sports injury	Connective Tissue Deficiency	Overuse
Main Treatment	Prolotherapy	Rest/NSAIDs
Ancillary Treatments	Nutrition/Dietary	Ice
Exercise	Encouraged	Discouraged
Treatment Objective	Strengthen Connective Tissue	Rest the Injury
End Result	Stronger Ligaments/Tendons	Weaker Tissue
Likelihood of Recurrence	Rare	Expected
Athletic Performance	Enhanced	Reduced

Athletes of the future will look at overuse syndrome as a connective tissue deficiency problem. Treatments such as the MEAT protocol, nutrition, and Prolotherapy will be used to strengthen the weakened structure.

As you can see, there is a big difference between viewing sports injuries as a connective tissue deficiency problem versus an overuse problem. Athletes love to train and need to train if they are going to excel in their sports. For the last 30 years, since the **RICE** protocol was first penned, athletes became hesitant to continually train hard because of fear of overuse syndrome. As we enter into the 21st century let's hope that a new era for the athlete will emerge, where an athlete can train as long and as hard as she/he desires. When an injury does occur, instead of suppressing the body's own inflammatory healing mechanisms, the sports medicine specialist of the future will give nutritional/dietary supplements that enhance healing and then administer treatments such as Neural Therapy and Prolotherapy to the injured site to optimize autonomic nervous function and stimulate fibroblastic proliferation. This is the way sports medicine should be practiced and is being practiced at places like Caring Medical in Oak Park, Illinois. The treatments used should stimulate the body to heal, not suppress it.

JUMPER'S KNEE: PATELLAR TENDINOSIS

To remain competitive, athletes today are subjected to intense and repetitive weight training, conditioning, and sport-specific drills. Often this training regimen occurs year-round without any breaks. This continual pounding of the pavement or gymnasium floor eventually takes its toll on the body. The athletes' knees are usually the first part of the body to become injured.

Jumper's knee is characterized as an "overuse injury" causing pathological changes in the distal parts of the extensor system of the knee joint, namely the quadriceps and patellar tendon (patellar ligament). As you will soon see, it is not an inflammatory condition, but a degenerative one.

93

SIDE VIEW OF THE KNEE

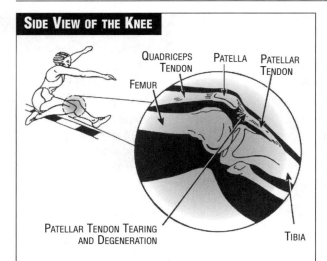

See Figure 6-19: Patellar Tendonitis (Jumper's Knee)
Sports such as volleyball and basketball require a lot of acceleration, deceleration, jumping, and landing. These actions concentrate a tremendous stress on the quadriceps muscle and patellar tendon of the knee making them prone to injury.

Reprinted by permission from G.H. Guten, 1991, Play Healthy, Stay Healthy *(Champaign, IL: Human Kinetics), p. 134.*

Jumper's knee is a clinical entity most commonly found in athletes who habitually place excessive strain on the extensor system of their knees, with numerous jumps or long periods of running during their athletic activities. *(See Figure 6-19.)* The high frequency of jumper's knee in volleyball players was first noticed by Maurizio in 1963.[33] Ferretti, who was a volleyball player himself, carried out an epidemiological study. The results of the study showed that jumper's knee accounted for 28 percent of all sports-related injuries in volleyball, and that 40 percent of top-level volleyball players suffer from this syndrome at least once during their athletic career.[34] A high incidence of jumper's knee was also noticed in other athletic activities, primarily in the so-called jumping sports such as the high jump, the long jump, the triple jump, and basketball.[35,36] Soccer players, weight lifters, hockey players, bicyclists, and skaters also experience jumper's knee, but to a lesser degree.[37] Jumper's knee can also develop in athletes who habitually run for long periods of time, as in long-distance runners.[38]

It is interesting to note how each athlete responds differently to the same stresses. For example, some develop jumper's knee while others remain symptom-free even though the athletes are participating in the same sport, playing in the same position on the team, and are placed under the same repeated mechanical stresses.[39] Something is inherent in certain people that makes them more prone to developing jumper's knee.

Various types of jumps are the main athletic activities that substantially increase the amount of mechanical strain placed upon the knee extensory system. These consist of both sudden and strongly performed jumps from a stationary position, as in performing a block in volleyball, and jumps taken while running, as in the long and high jumps. It is important to note that the quadriceps tendon bears the maximal amount of mechanical strain during the deceleration phase of the landing at which time the quadriceps femoris muscle is overcoming the force of gravity with its eccentric contraction.[40] *(See Figure*

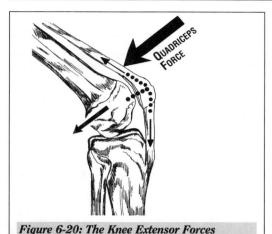

Figure 6-20: The Knee Extensor Forces
Jumping occurs because of the tremendous force exerted by the quadriceps tendon. It is this structure and the patellar tendon that become injured in "jumpers knee."
Used by permission from Nike's **Common Running Injuries • Sport Research Review,** *March/April, 1989.*

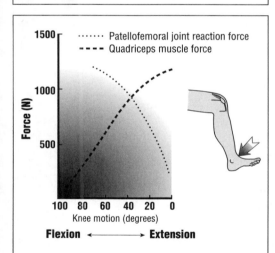

Figure 6-21: The Amount of Extensor Forces at Varying Degrees of Knee Range of Motion
Jumping sporting activities put tremendous forces on the quadriceps muscle.
Used with permission from V. H. Frankel and M. Nordin: **Basic Biomechanics of the Skeletal System,** *Philadelphia, 1980, Lea & Febriger.*

6-20.) When eccentrically contracting at landing, the quadriceps tendon force can exceed 1,000 Newtons. *(See Figure 6-21.)*

Studies have shown that the training method used by the athletes has no significant bearing on the development of jumper's knee. The amount of habitual activity played a much more causative role in the development of jumper's knee.[41] Determining which athlete will develop jumper's knee is likely related to the presence of a malalignment in the lower extremity. From a clinical standpoint, the orientation of the lower extremity is determined by the value of the angle of the quadriceps femoris muscle or the Q-angle. *(See Figure 6-22.)* The normal value of this angle is up to 10 degrees in males and no more than 15 degrees in females. The Q-angle is slightly greater in females because of the width of the female pelvis. Pecina and associates reported a significant correlation between a pathological Q-angle and the development of jumper's knee.[37] Ferretti and associates reported a 50-percent presence of pathological values for the Q-angle in their total sample.[42]

Measuring Q-angles is great, but generally the volleyball players who come to our office do not care about their Q-angles, they just want to get rid of their pain. The pain typically starts out as a pain in the knee after a game or practice. Then it begins to appear at the beginning of activity, improves with the activity, but starts hurting like the dickens after the sporting event. Eventually the pain becomes constant and the athlete must cease playing, unless, of course, they receive Prolotherapy.

The pain is always related to the quadriceps or the patellar tendon, typically at the attachment site of the patellar tendon to the patella. This area is exquisitely tender; therefore, it is very easy to elicit a positive jump sign during the physical examination. Pecina and associates reported the appearance of pain at the junction of the quadriceps tendon to the base of the patella in 20 percent of their patients; at the insertion of the patellar tendon to the tibial tuberosity in 12 percent; and at the insertion site of the patellar tendon at the tip of the patella in 68 percent of the athletes suffering from jumper's knee.[43] *(See Figure 6-23.)*

The pain of jumper's knee is first characterized by a well-localized, dull ache of insidious onset, and the athlete has no recollection of a specific traumatic event. Complaints of weakness or giving way are common, although true locking, clicking, or knee effusion are rarely seen. With continued participation in the sport and no Prolotherapy, the pain may begin to appear at the beginning of practice, disappear after "warming up," and frequently reappear after completion of the activity. As the degenerative process continues, eventually, without rest, the pain becomes constant and remains during and after activity. Athletic performance is drastically impaired. It is not uncommon for athletes to lose vast amounts of playing time because of jumper's knee. *(See Figure 6-24.)* The pain often becomes constant. Jumping, landing, climbing stairs, sitting for prolonged periods of time with the knee flexed, and, in more severe cases, just walking will exacerbate the symptoms.

Increasing amounts of evidence are accumulating indicating that jumper's knee involves a chronic deteriorating or degenerative condition of the patellar and quadriceps tendon, primarily at its fibro-osseous junction. Ferretti and

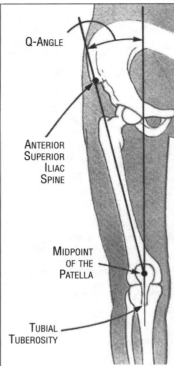

Figure 6-22: The Q-Angle
The larger the Q-angle, the more likely an athlete will get "jumper's knee" and need Prolotherapy.

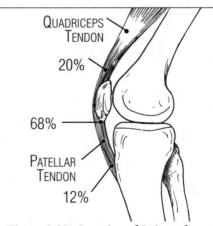

Figure 6-23: Location of Pain and Injury in Jumper's Knee
Jumper's knee involves injury to the patellar tendon and/or quadriceps tendon.

associates noted that the basic pathological changes develop on the insertion sites of the quadriceps tendon and patellar tendon to the patella and tibial tuberosity.[44] The changes consist of a thickening of the transition cartilages between the tendon and bone, the appearance of cystic cavities, and the loss of the border between the two transition cartilages. These changes occur at the fibro-osseous junction where the tendon attaches to the bone. Further research has shown that histopathological changes are also evident in the tendon structure.[45] For this reason, it is best to look at jumper's knee as an enthesis (insertional tendinopathy) as well as a change in the tendon structure (tendinosis).

Athletes with recalcitrant knee pain sometimes accept surgery as a treatment option. One good thing about surgery is that the physicians can actually see what is going on in the knee because they cut it open to look at it. Unfortunately, the end results are often very bad for the athletes. The surgery involves debriding (removing) all of the degenerated tissue. The athlete is typically restricted from athletic competition for four to six months, with the symptoms of knee pain often persisting for eight to 12 months after the surgery.[46] The deterioration in the tissues typically depends upon the duration of the symptoms. Regardless of the duration of the symptoms, the fundamental defect in chronic jumper's knee is **degeneration—not inflammation**. Bassett and associates performed an in-depth study on the pathology involved in jumper's knee. Mucoid degeneration of collagen with focal loss of staining was seen in patients with symptoms of less than six months' duration, when tissue was examined under the microscope. The finely-organized appearance of normal collagen was lost. *(See Figures 6-25a and 6-25b.)* Of note was the lack of inflammatory cells. Further fibrocartilaginous formation and portions of dense fibrous tissue, with degeneration and some

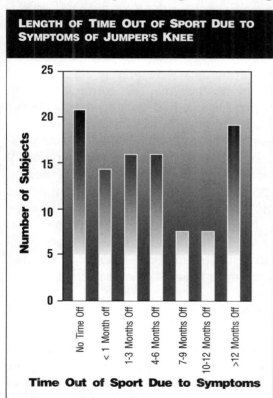

LENGTH OF TIME OUT OF SPORT DUE TO SYMPTOMS OF JUMPER'S KNEE

Number of Subjects vs. *Time Out of Sport Due to Symptoms*

Categories: No Time Off, < 1 Month off, 1-3 Months Off, 4-6 Months Off, 7-9 Months Off, 10-12 Months Off, >12 Months Off

Figure 6-24: Time Out of Sport Due to Symptoms from Jumper's Knee
Knee pain in jumpers should be evaluated by a Prolotherapist, otherwise, sporting activities will be curtailed by necessity.

Adapted from: *A cross sectional study of 100 athletes with Jumper's Knee*, by J. L. Cook, et al., British Journal of Sports Medicine, *London, 1997; 31:332-336, BMJ Publishing Group. Used by permission.*

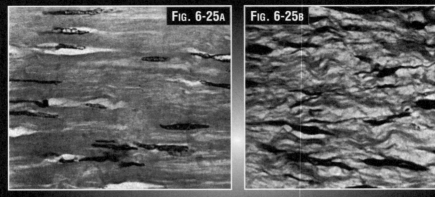

Figure 6-25: Normal and Post-Surgical Tendon
Figure 6-25a (on left) shows the normal appearance of a patellar tendon. Figure 6-25b (on right) shows a histologic specimen at surgical exploration in a 19 year old basketball player ("Jumper's knee"). Note the loss of the normal tendon architecture and staining characteristics. The slides show degeneration with ___no___ inflammatory component.
Slides used by permission A. Colosimo, Jumper's Knee, *Orthopedic Review, 19:148, 1990.*

calcified cartilage, were noted when symptoms were present for six to 12 months. Myxomatous tissue (a group of mesenchymal cells forming a benign growth) was frequently found. Further disorganization, together with the formation of chondroid matrices and some spicules of bone were seen when symptoms lasted longer than one year.[46,47] You do not have to know what myxomatous tissue is to know that it is bad. What is mucoid degeneration of collagen? Who knows? But it sure sounds bad! Sometimes all of this medical terminology becomes overwhelming. Mucoid degeneration of collagen occurs when tendon tissue and the fibro-osseous junction deteriorate. This is the same process that occurs during prolonged joint immobilization. The tendons, ligaments, muscles, cartilage, and bone begin deteriorating because the normal strong organized collagen tissue that makes up these structures becomes disorganized and is replaced by various forms of scar tissue. It is that simple.

TREATMENTS FOR JUMPER'S KNEE
CORTICOSTEROID INJECTIONS

A common question is whether a cortisone injection into this area is a good idea. No, it is a bad idea. It is probably the cause of much of the deterioration. Andrea Ferretti and associates at the University of Roma in Rome, Italy, studied the histological findings in 18 patients who underwent surgical repair for jumper's knee. The patients consisted of nine volleyball players, three basketball players, one high jumper, one soccer player, one ballet dancer, and three unaccounted for. The surgery involved drilling some holes into the patella at the exact site of the pain, as well as a lateral release surgery to help the patella track better. The tendon and bone tissues were sent to pathology for analysis. During the surgery, 15 of the tendons appeared to be in perfect condition according to the surgeons and three tendons had noticeable degeneration visible to the naked eye.

The three cases of visible tendon necrosis (degeneration) occurred in patients who had received repeated local injections of corticosteroids. The physicians stated "…owing to the absence of alterations of the patellar tendon in all the other cases of 'jumper's knee' that did not receive local injections of steroids, we speculated that the abnormalities found in the patellar tendon were secondary to the jeopardizing effect of the cortisone rather than primary."[48]

The above data is amazing. When cortisone was given, obvious tendon deterioration was observed by the surgeons. Perhaps all of the chronic tendinoses are just due to the treatments the athletes are receiving and not due to the actual sporting activities. Cortisone leads to massive tendon deterioration. These observations are very interesting. We will let you ponder them for a while.

In all the cases, Dr. Ferretti found degeneration of the fibro-osseous junction where the patellar tendon attached to the tibia and patella. They noted "…our histologic findings seem to indicate that abnormalities of the patellar osteotendinous junction either of the quadricepital or the patellar tendon are present in 'jumper's knee.' The main abnormalities found were pseudocystic cavities at the borderline between mineralized fibrocartilage and bone, increased thickness of the fibrocartilage, myxomatosis, and hyaline metaplasia of the fibrocartilage."[48]

Of the 18 surgical patients, six experienced excellent results, five had good results, and seven had poor results. In the study, the excellent result rate with surgery for jumper's knee was 33 percent. There is a better way.

A MORE NATURAL, SUCCESSFUL APPROACH: PROLOTHERAPY

As we have just seen, numerous studies have documented definite degenerative pathology in the patellar tendon. This type of degeneration also occurs in other chronic sports injuries such as Achilles tendon and rotator cuff problems. The problem is that researchers are forgetting "the cortisone factor." They see degenerative tissue and blame it on overtraining or overuse. In other words, the athlete is to blame for the development of the chronic pain. They are supposedly training too hard, causing their Achilles tendons to deteriorate. Does this make sense to you? We don't think so.

Neither the American Medical Association, the American Association of Orthopedic Surgeons, nor the Food and Drug Administration has evaluated the statement we are about to make. As U.S. citizens, however, under the first amendment of the U.S. Constitution, we can hereby declare that a good portion of the degenerative tendon tissue found on pathological or histological studies is caused by a physician directly injecting cortisone, or one of its derivatives, directly or indirectly around tendons. The above study confirmed this.

Ultrasound and histology data were obtained in a recent study done on 100 athletes with jumper's knee. The researchers found that 48 of the subjects developed initial symptoms of jumper's knee before the age of 20. Symptoms prevented 33 of the athletes from participating in their sports for more than six months, and 18 of these were sidelined for more than 12 months. Ultrasound studies of the patellar tendon showed a characteristic hypoechoic region at the junction of the inferior pole of the patella and the deep surface of the patellar tendon. Histopathological examination showed separation and disruption of collagen fibers on polarization light microscopy and an increase in mucoid ground substance consistent with damage of tendon collagen without inflammation.[49] In lay language, the histopathological examination of the tendon lesions showed tendon degeneration or microtears, or both, rather than inflammatory cells. In other words, the pain is caused by degeneration not by inflammation. The questions you should now ask yourselves are: "Why then do I keep getting anti-inflammatories and why do I keep swallowing them?" These are good questions!

You are, hopefully, beginning to understand the reason for the writing of this book. Do you now see why NSAIDs, cortisone shots, and a large part of what is called "sports medicine" could be called "sports degeneration"?

Follow these simple instructions when you are injured and you will most certainly accelerate degeneration and stop the healing process:

1. When injured, put massive amounts of ice on the site.

2. To decrease the swelling elevate the limb, compress it with tape, and even better yet, wrap the ice in the tape so you can cool and compress the area at the same time.

3. Make sure you rest the injured limb until seen in follow-up in one week.

4. Make sure you take an anti-inflammatory medication, as this will dramatically increase the effects of this protocol.

5. Upon follow-up in one week, when you still have pain, a cortisone injection will be given into the area.

6. Continue the rest and inactivity for two more weeks. Put a brace on the injured body part to add stability.

7. Upon follow-up in three weeks, you should notice instability in the joint. The joint should be loose and weakened. Exquisite tenderness at the injury site confirms that you have been successful in permanently stopping the healing of the injury. Congratulations!

NO INFLAMMATION PRESENT

We are sorry, but we have one more study. The studies need to be in this book, so you know that the things we are saying are supported by respected researchers from around the world, their studies being presented in some of the most well-respected medical and sports medicine journals around the world. People other than the authors and contributors to this book believe these tenets.

MRIs, histological evaluation, and surgical treatments were done on nine patients with recalcitrant knee pain at the Ohio State University Sports

Medicine Center.[50] The athletes were all diagnosed with jumper's knee. MRI scans revealed abnormalities in all of the patellar tendons and histological analysis confirmed evidence of tendon degeneration. The specimens showed evidence of angioblastic tendinosis revealing disorganized collagen and hyaline degeneration. Most noticeably absent from all of the specimens were acute inflammatory cells. Chronic sports injuries do not require any more anti-inflaming because not even one cell is left to anti-inflame!

KARLA: JUMPER'S KNEE AND STILL JUMPING

Karla was one of those sturdy athletes. She came to our missionary clinic, Beulah Land Natural Medicine Clinic in Thebes, Illinois, with severe knee pain. "I've had knee problems since seventh grade," she explained. She had been playing volleyball since seventh grade. "My knees are terrible. I'm on athletic scholarship for volleyball and it just kills to jump." You see Karla was the middle hitter—the tall lady in the middle who does most of the spiking. She needed to play well because her college educational expenses depended on it!

Karla had classic jumper's knee, exhibiting significant pain with contraction of the quadriceps/patellar tendons. Both of these tendon attachments were injected (lucky her). I (Ross) recently telephoned her regarding her status. "Karla, how are you doing?" "What? Who is this?" (I apparently woke her up. Isn't everybody up at 6:30 a.m.?) Then I thought, "Is she in the same time zone as we are? My fears vanished when I realized that she was in our time zone, but that it was just 6:30 a.m. and she was asleep. (Come on, get up!) I explained who I was and why I was calling, but she was not too impressed. Perhaps she was still partly asleep. We may never know.

At least Karla gave us these words, "I definitely felt improvement with the treatment. My pain is less. I finished the season, so I have a break now." I ended with, "So, I'll see you at the next clinic?" Then she said, "No, I'm just too busy with summer school and everything." I asked, "Are you playing volleyball next season?" She replied, "Oh, yes, middle hitter." The conversation continued for a few more minutes, but again we were left with that same question. Why do athletes continue to play with pain, when they know that pain is always telling them that something is wrong? For Karla, it was her tendons. Until she strengthens them with Prolotherapy, they will continue to deteriorate to the point where she will be advised to see a physician with something bigger than a syringe and needle, desiring to plunge it into her knee. We suspect that when that day occurs, Karla will remember her doctor-friend who woke her up that one early morning on the phone. When we see her then we will smile and politely say, "Prolotherapy anyone?"

KNEE PAIN: THE NEMESIS FOR THOSE WHO LOVE TO JUMP

We all see those pieces of cloth wrapped around the athletes' knees at all athletic levels—from Little Leaguers to professionals. It is our hope that after reading this book, basketball players and those who play jumping sports will realize that nothing is a substitute for a strong joint, not even tape of the most secure kind. The strength of the joint is primarily dependent on the integrity of its ligaments.

The knee is surrounded by strong ligaments and contains the largest ligament in the human body (patellar ligament). The knee is uniquely vulnerable to injury because of its precarious location midway between the hip and ankle, and

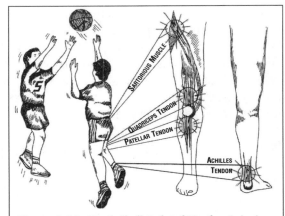

Figure 6-26: Basketball-Related Tendon Injuries
Jumping sports are notorious for tearing up tendons, especially of the lower extremities.

because of the tremendous forces transmitted from the ground through the knee to the hip. It is also the site of attachment of many tendons and muscles, so it is vulnerable to both acute traumatic injuries as well as overuse syndromes. *(See Figure 6-26.)* The medial knee compartment is more constrained than the lateral compartment because of the osseous, meniscal, and ligamentous morphology. This may explain the greater prevalence of medial knee injuries.

PES ANSERINUS TENDONITIS IN BASKETBALL PLAYERS

Pes anserinus tendonitis is a frequent cause of medial knee pain in athletes who participate in sports involving a lot of running, pivoting, jumping, and sudden decelerations, all of which describe the game of basketball. The athlete generally complains of pain in the medial compartment of the knee when running, cut-

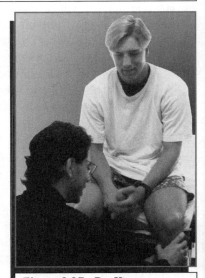

Figure 6-27: Dr. Hauser Examining the Pes Anserinus Area for a "Positive Jump Sign"
Junior tennis star Gregg Hill unfortunately had a lot of "Positive Jump Signs..."

ting, or kicking the ball. The pain can be reproduced by palpating the tibial insertion area of the pes anserinus tendons and eliciting a positive jump sign *(See Figure 6-27.)* Passive external rotation and resisted internal rotation during the flexion-extension movements of the knee can also reproduce the pain.

The pes anserinus is the combined tendinous insertion of the sartorius, gracilis, and semitendinosus tendons at their attachments to the tibia. The

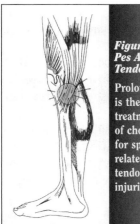

Figure 6-28: Pes Anserinus Tendonitis

Prolotherapy is the treatment of choice for sports-related tendon injuries.

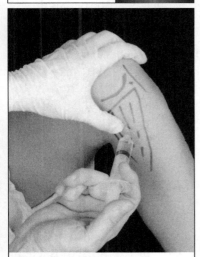

Figure 6-29: Injection of the Pes Anserinus

Prolotherapy is very effective at treating pes anserinus tendon injury, a common cause of chronic knee pain in athletes.

pes anserinus bursa lies between this insertion and the bone. Athletes tell Prolotherapists that the orthopedist injected cortisone shots in the painful area because the diagnosis of bursitis was given. Bursitis is extremely rare. Extreme pain, significant swelling, and redness characterize a true bursitis. The area is so painful that the patient cannot even handle light touch to the area. When asked if this is an adequate description of the pain, the usual response is the following, "Oh, no doctor, I have pain that comes and goes and gets worse with exercise." This is not indicative of a bursitis, but a tendonitis. The tendon becomes inflamed because it is trying to repair itself. The best approach is to continue to promote the natural healing process, not stop it with various anti-inflammatory treatments.

Typical treatments by traditional team physicians for pes anserinus tendonitis include the **RICE** protocol, anti-inflammatories, and cortisone injections. These can potentially cause weakening of the tendons. A better approach is Prolotherapy, which is very effective at strengthening the pes anserine tendons. *(See Figure 6-28.)* Once this is done the athlete is usually cured of the medial knee pain. The medial side of the knee is much stronger, which leads to enhanced athletic performance overall.

Prolotherapy to the pes anserinus tendon area is one of the most rewarding injections to perform. This is because the treatment of this area takes less than one minute and the results are often instantaneous. *(See Figure 6-29.)* A good example of this was when the host/producer of the national cable show *COPE*, Dr. Karen Hayter, was treated live on the air of *Your Health Matters*, a national radio show.

We were in Dallas, Texas, promoting *Prolo Your Pain Away!* and were on the *COPE* show with host Doug Kaufmann. Karen was producing the show and Doug was acting host, as he does most Fridays. Karen was hobbling around and told us how her orthopedist said she had arthritis and would soon need a knee replacement. She was given a brace and some NSAIDs. Ross examined her, right then and there, and found that she had excellent range of motion. A diagnosis of arthritis in a person with good range of motion in the knees but a wobbly gait can only mean one thing. He poked on her pes anserinus area and she let out a yell! She displayed a good example of a positive jump sign.

She was then given the good news and the bad news. The good news was that her problem could be fixed, but the bad news was that the fix involved a needle. Karen said she would have to think about it. After the show, we agreed to treat her live on the air during Doug's radio show the next morning.

Karen arrived promptly at 9:00 a.m. We had been on the air since 7:00 a.m., so Ross had a little time to be nervous, because he had been promoting Prolotherapy on Doug's show for two hours and now the moment of truth had come. He knew Prolotherapy was going to help Karen, but he just did not know if she was going to scream when the injections were given.

They talked to the audience live on the air as he examined her. He cleaned the area with alcohol and then plunged the 27-gauge needle into the pes anserinus tendons and gave Karen shot after shot. Fortunately, Doug had Karen gagged so she could not say anything. No, Karen did great, and in a couple of minutes it was all over. Within five minutes, 50 percent of her pain was gone. He did a few more shots and, within the hour, Karen was over 90 percent better. She was getting out of her chair without any pain. She left that hour without a brace and without the need for NSAIDs. She was also grateful because she was going on a guided tour of Israel the next week. The trip included walking the Jericho trail that Jesus walked—all 17 miles of it. Karen was able to walk all 17 miles without any pain. The tour almost killed her, but her knees felt great.

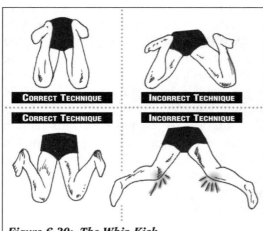

Figure 6-30: The Whip Kick
If done improperly, the whip kick places increased pressures on the medial side of the knee, injuring the medial collateral ligament. This condition is justifiably called "Breaststroker's Knee."

BREASTSTROKER'S KNEE

In 1974, Kennedy and Hawkins conducted a survey on the incidence of injuries to various parts of the musculoskeletal system of swimmers, and noticed that a high percentage of breaststroke swimmers complained of pain in the medial knee.[51] This condition has been termed breaststroker's knee, although further studies by Vizsoly (et al) on a population of 391 competitive swimmers showed that breaststroker's knee was diagnosed in 56 out of 77 breaststroke swimmers (73 percent), but also in 153 out of 314 swimmers (48 percent) who used either the freestyle, backstroke, or butterfly stroke.[52]

The condition is primarily seen in breaststrokers because of the whip kick. Much of the speed in the breaststroke comes from the whip kick. *(See Figure 6-30.)* Kennedy and Hawkins' initial paper reported that the condition was caused by weakness in the medial collateral ligament, resulting from repeated stretching during breaststroke swimming. In their opinion, the stretching of the ligament was caused by the extension part of the "whip kick," accompanied by an excessive valgus stress on the knee joint and the outward rotation of the leg in the final phase of the stroke.

The medial collateral ligament is the main supporting structure on the medial side of the knee; it is also called the tibial collateral ligament. Tension in the ligament increases as the knee moves from flexion to extension. This is exactly what happens during the kicking motion of the whip kick during breaststroke swimming. All the force is generated right at, directly on, bulls-eye hit to the medial collateral ligament.

Different authors point to different areas on the ligament that are causing the pain, but the main point is that, uniformly the pain-producing structure in breaststroker's knee is a laxity or sprain of the medial collateral ligament.[53, 54]

The cause of breaststroker's knee, according to traditional orthopedic sports medicine, is due to improper technique of doing the whip kick.[52, 55] For this reason, biomechanical factors are adjusted and the athlete is told to take time off from the sport. Some authors have suggested breaststrokers take at least two months off per year to allow the medial collateral ligament to heal.[51]

Most competitive athletes we have met do not care to take two months off from their sports. The swimmer with breaststroker's knee comes in complaining of medial knee pain, especially while swimming. There is severe pain upon palpation of both attachments of the medial collateral ligament. This then meets all the criteria for the athlete to receive Prolotherapy and makes him/her an excellent candidate. The Prolotherapy criteria are these: desire to get better, willingness to get shots, pain emanating from a ligament or tendon, and the pain can be reproduced in the office. Athletes with breaststroker's knee meet all of these criteria and the condition responds beautifully to Prolotherapy. *(See Figure 6-31.)*

After a swimmer receives Prolotherapy to the injured ligament, the physician urges them to train harder, not rest. Prolotherapy can make that ligament tremendously strong so the athlete never has to think about injuring it. Three to six sessions of

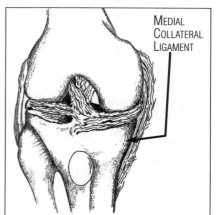

MEDIAL COLLATERAL LIGAMENT

Figure 6-31: Breaststroker's Knee

The whip kick in the breaststroke can cause injury to the medial collateral ligament. Prolotherapy to this ligament is often curative for the condition.

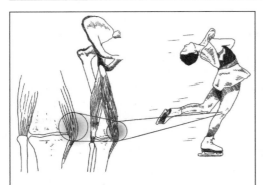

Figure 6-32: Hamstring Syndrome in a Skater
Any sport that involves a lot of running or leg movement inevitably makes the athlete prone to this condition.

Prolotherapy are generally required to resolve breaststroker's knee. Ross' favorite saying is "No matter what happens in life, no matter how bad the knee pain, you can always Prolo Your Pain Away!"

HAMSTRING SYNDROME: HAMSTRING ORIGIN TENDONITIS

Hamstring syndrome is a condition that affects muscles of the posterior thigh, primarily the hamstring muscles, which are the semitendinosis, semimembranosus, and biceps femoris muscles. *(See Figure 6-32.)* This condition frequently occurs in sprinters, hurdlers, skaters, and both long and high jumpers, but can also be found in other athletes, especially those who engage in rapid acceleration and short intense sprinting, such as hockey, baseball, football, and soccer players, as well as hurdlers, tennis players, and others.[56]

Most authors today agree that the basic causative reason for the development of hamstring syndrome is the muscle strength imbalance between the hamstring muscle group and the quadriceps femoris muscles. The normal biomechanics of the lower extremity depend on the smoothly-coordinated reciprocal action between the quadriceps and the hamstring muscle group. Studies have indicated that the hamstring muscles should have at least 60 percent of the strength of the quadriceps in athletes. This is often not the case with the hamstrings, which have 40 percent or less of the strength of the quadriceps, especially in athletes involved in running sports.[57,58] A 10 percent or greater muscle strength deficit between the two sides is also thought to be a predisposition for hamstring strain.[57]

The athlete with hamstring syndrome generally complains of buttock pain that radiates down the back of the thigh. The pain typically increases during the performance of forcible or sudden movements, which stretch the hamstring muscles (i.e., in sprinting or hurdling). Another characteristic complaint is pain felt while sitting, such as while driving a car or sitting during lectures. The pain is often relentless, causing the person to change positions or stand up for relief.

During the physical examination, **My Reproducibility Instrument**, the thumb, can reproduce the athlete's pain. Severe pain occurs when the examiner's thumb presses on the ischial tuberosity where the hamstring muscles originate.

Traditional treatments include hamstring stretches, because tight hamstrings have also been implicated in causing the condition. The athlete is encouraged to rest the area, and reduce inflammation with ice and NSAIDs.[57] Remember, these are traditional recommendations, not ours!

Physiotherapy/kinesiotherapy is definitely needed for the athlete with this condition, to improve hamstring length and strength. It is important that the traditional hamstring stretches not be done, as these just make the tight hamstrings tighter. The ischial tuberosity fibro-osseous junction is injected with Prolotherapy because the weakness felt by the athlete involves the origin of the hamstring muscles. Prolotherapy strengthens this area, which is the precise area of weakness in hamstring syndrome or hamstring tendonitis. After three to six treatments, the buttock pain and posterior thigh pain is typically relieved. If the problem resides within the hamstring muscle itself, massage and myofascial release therapy is done as well. Neural Therapy injections to the muscle belly and surrounding structures can also be given to relax the muscle and improve healing.

PROLOTHERAPY IS CRUCIAL FOR ATHLETES WITH CRUCIATE LIGAMENT INJURY.

Throughout this book is information on why athletes with cruciate ligament injuries need Prolotherapy. Here is a synopsis:

- *Cruciate injury leads to arthritis.*
- *Cruciate surgery produces sub-optimal results.*
- *Surgically-repaired knees still end up with accelerated arthritis.*
- *Prolotherapy can repair all the structures in the knee.*
- *Prolotherapy gets the injured structures stronger.*
- *Prolotherapy recovery time is days—compared to weeks..*

(See Figure 6-33.)

PROLOTHERAPY VERSUS KNEE SURGERY

	PROLOTHERAPY	KNEE SURGERY
Stimulates repair	Yes	No
Increases collagen strength	Yes	No
Arthritis risk	Decreased	Increased
Return to sport	Quick	Slow
Rehabilitation time	Short	Long
Exercise	Encouraged	Cautious
Anesthesia required	No	Yes
Cost	Hundreds	Thousands
Time involved in procedure	Minutes	Hours
Instruments used	Thin needles	Massive Scopes/Scapels

Figure 6-33: Prolotherapy versus Knee Surgery

Prolotherapy has many advantages over knee surgery; so why are so many athletes receiving arthroscopies?

KNEE INJURIES AND ALPINE SKIING

The anterior cruciate ligament (ACL) sprain is the most common injury seen in skiing. An estimated 100,000 anterior cruciate ligaments are injured each year due to skiing accidents.[59] Because the ski produces a long lever arm, the anterior cruciate ligaments may be injured through many possible mechanisms. Catching a ski tip in heavy snow produces an external rotation/valgus stress on the knee, which may tear the medial collateral ligament as well. Forced hyperextension may occur during deceleration when skiing from a fast, packed surface onto heavy untracked snow. The anterior cruciate ligament is the normal structure that restricts hyperextension of the knee.

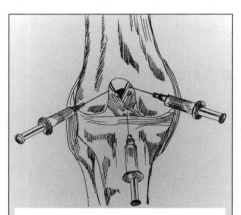

Figure 6-34: Prolotherapy of the Knee
Because of the propensity of skiers to sustain ACL and PCL injuries, rolotherapy should replace arthroscopy as the skier's best friend.

ACL INJURY

Deficiency or laxity in the ACL leads to recurrent instability and eventual arthritis. Fetto and Marshall reported in 1980 that non-operative treatment leads to a degree of functional limitation in 92 percent of patients. The frequency of unstable "giving-way" episodes of the knee increased over time.[62] Many other reports have also documented that if the ACL does not heal properly or completely, the ability to ski long-term will likely decline and the athlete will experience significant knee instability, a continual feeling of the knee "giving way," and a long-term likelihood of the development of proliferative arthritis in the knee. [59-61, 63-65]

The best treatment for the athlete with a ligament tear in the knee is Prolotherapy. *(See Figure 6-34.)* Most ligament tears in the knee, as well as other areas of the body, are typically not complete tears. Even severe acute tears respond well to Prolotherapy because the treatment initiates the inflammatory healing cascade to regenerate new ligament tissue. The athlete who does not receive proper treatment for an ACL tear after the initial injury, will regret it for a long time. One hundred thousand skiers injure this ligament every year. This is the main stabilizing ligament of the knee. The non-healing of this one ligament is probably responsible for the majority of total knee replacements done in the United States. The choice is simple for the skier, Prolotherapy today or total knee replacement tomorrow.

PCL INJURY

Regardless of which knee ligament is injured, arthritis and degenerative changes will follow if the knee is left untreated or improperly treated. Even an

108

isolated posterior cruciate ligament-deficient knee is fraught with long-term degenerative changes and pain.[66] The posterior cruciate ligament (PCL) is injured in skiers when they collide with a fixed object, smashing the front of the tibia bone. If this injury does not heal properly, the skier is again left with an unstable knee. The knee requires all of its ligaments to function properly. If even one ligament is sacrificed, as often occurs during arthroscopy, detrimental consequences result because God put each and every ligament in the knee for a reason.

In one study, 40 patients with posterior cruciate ligament injuries (30 of the 40 were sports-related) were followed-up at four to six years after initial injury.[67] Sixty-five percent of the patients revealed that their activity level after injury was limited. Forty-nine percent stated that the involved knee had not fully recovered despite rehabilitation. Ninety percent complained of knee pain with activity and 43 percent complained of problems with walking. The x-rays of the knees without a normal PCL were horrible. The radiographic degenerative changes increased over time after the injury. Of the patients examined more than four years after injury, only 12 percent had normal x-rays of their knees. Sixty-five percent showed extensive degenerative changes.

WHAT ABOUT SURGERY?

These facts are horrible and should scare athletes to death. Six years after a single ligament injury, 65 percent of the people are still limiting their activities and 90 percent have pain in their knees. Sixty percent of the knees appeared "shot" on the x-ray film. The amazing thing is that the PCL is not even the main ligament in the knee! People often say, "Well doctor, if it is so bad, shouldn't I just get surgery?" No! Why receive surgery when Prolotherapy can stimulate the exact ligaments to regenerate? A tendon graft or artificial graft will never totally simulate the original ligament tissue. Ligament tissue and tendon tissue are different.

Surgery typically involves suturing the ligament ends together or making a new ligament by grafting the patellar tendon tissue to where the ligament should be located. When a patellar tendon graft is used, it does not take on all of the biochemical properties of the posterior cruciate ligament.[68] This has been documented histologically, by examining the tissue under the microscope. If true ligament tissue is not the final result, then the outcome cannot be very good. In one study of 53 patients seen eight years after surgery, 66 percent were at the same intensity level as they were prior to the injury, but 34 percent were not back to normal. Seventy percent of the patients had stable knees, but 78 percent suffered degenerative changes in the knees. Surgery helps some people, but a good percentage still go on to have problems and degenerative changes in their knees.[69]

For this reason, many athletes are regenerating their damaged knee ligaments with Prolotherapy. Prolotherapy stimulates the body to repair the damaged ligaments. In regards to the posterior and anterior cruciate ligaments, since these are intra-articular ligaments, the injections are done to the inside of the knee joint. Both ends of the ligaments are typically injected. If the person is an athlete and it is vital to get back to training, then the treatments are done once every one to three weeks. For people with chronic knee pain and laxity in the knee, Prolotherapy is typically given once per month to every six weeks, to allow enough time for ligament growth. After three to six sessions, the cruciate ligaments are generally strong again and the knee has regained its stability. Once this happens, the athlete's knee feels stronger so athletic performance is enhanced. Even more important is that the degenerative process stops and the long-term prognosis for the athlete is excellent.

POSTEROLATERAL KNEE PAIN: THINK POPLITEUS MUSCLE AND POPLITEOFIBULAR LIGAMENT

Posterior knee pain in the athlete can originate from several soft tissue structures in the knee. If the athlete feels the knee is unstable, the pain may be coming from the cruciate ligaments, since these refer pain to the back of the knee. Posterior knee pain precipitated by acceleration or deceleration (e.g., downhill running, kicking, or sprinting) is likely to be semimembranosus or popliteus tendonitis. These can easily be differentiated because they attach on opposite sides of the knee. The popliteus muscle originates on the lateral part of the lateral femoral condyle. The popliteus muscle rotates the tibia medially when the thigh is fixed and the leg is free to move, as when sitting erect. During weight-bearing when the leg is fixed, this muscle rotates the femur laterally on the tibia to "unlock" the knee joint. *(See Figure 6-35.)*

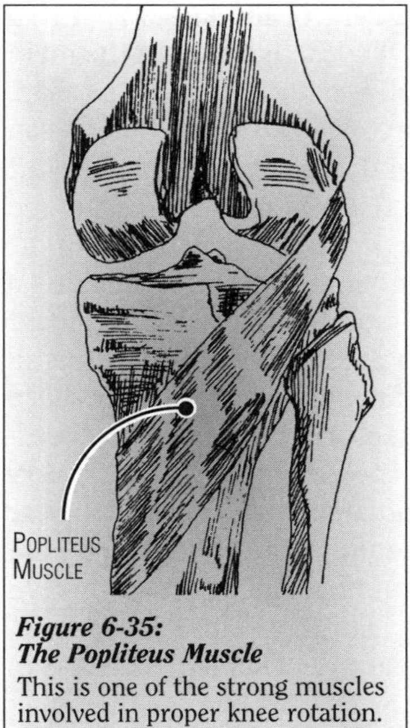

If the popliteus muscle is tender and palpation to this area reproduces the patient's pain, it is injected. If the muscle belly is the tender area, Neural Therapy will be given and kinesiotherapy ordered. If the origin of the muscle is tender on the femoral condyle, then this will be treated with Prolotherapy. Prolotherapy will start the proliferation of the muscle tissue and strengthen the origin. For many people this is all that is needed to relieve their posterior knee pain.

The popliteal muscle has a significant attachment to the fibula, the popliteofibular ligament. The lateral section of this is also called the ligament of Valois.[70] The popliteofibular ligament is important in resisting posterior translation and varus and external rotation of

Figure 6-35:
The Popliteus Muscle
This is one of the strong muscles involved in proper knee rotation.

Adapted from Total Body Training by Richard H. Dominguez, M.D., and Robert Gajda©1982. Used by permission.

POPLITEUS
MUSCLE

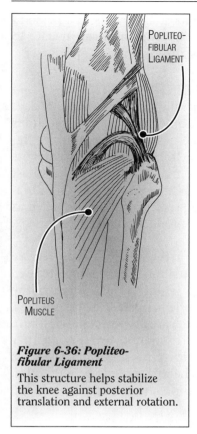

POPLITEO-
FIBULAR
LIGAMENT

POPLITEUS
MUSCLE

***Figure 6-36: Popliteo-
fibular Ligament***

This structure helps stabilize
the knee against posterior
translation and external rotation.

the knee.[71] *(See Figure 6-36.)* In other words, it is a key player in stabilizing the knee posteriorly and laterally. The order of stability on the lateral side of the knee when a person receives a blow to that side of the knee is as follows: the lateral collateral ligament fails first, followed by the popliteofibular ligament, and then the muscle belly of the popliteus. The mean maximal force to failure of the popliteofibular ligament approaches 425N compared with 750N for the lateral collateral ligament.[72] Any time an athlete sustains a varus stress on the knee, as occurs during a hockey match or a tackle in football, injury to the popliteofibular ligament should be investigated.

The athlete with an injury to the popliteofibular ligament has point tenderness behind the fibular head. Prolotherapy to this area is effective at stimulating the growth of normal ligament tissue. Once the popliteofibular ligament is thickened and of normal strength, the posterolateral knee pain subsides. Generally, the knee also feels more stable. The athlete is grateful for this and can continue playing hockey or any other sport.

RUNNING AND JOGGING

When we run, our foot is only on the ground for 40 percent of the time. When you compare this with walking, you find that we are on both feet at least 60 percent of the entire stride. The contact with the ground and the tremendous forces generated cause the injuries to occur. In a recent study, it was found that no matter what shoes the runners wore, the injuries and complaints stayed the same. These statistics showed that 28 percent of runners had shin splints, 25 percent had knee pain, 21 percent had calf pain, while only 15 percent had injured their ankles. What is most amazing is that 81 percent of all runners questioned had some pain somewhere at some time.

When we examine what is really happening in the runner, the problems become clear. The first obvious problem is that we produce shock when our foot pounds into the ground with tremendous forces being generated. The second is the inability of the body to dissipate the shock, and the third is the extreme movement of the joints and ligaments while running.

Excessive pronation—especially while running—can be the underlying culprit, causing chronic knee, hip, or back pain. *(See Figure 6-37.)* Sometimes

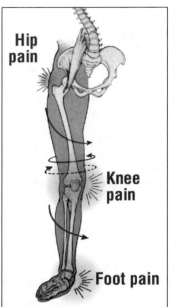

Hip pain

Knee pain

Foot pain

Excessive pronation

Figure 6-37: The Ankle Bone's Connected to the Foot Bone...

Laxity in the ankle and foot ligaments can cause not only foot pain, but lead to knee and hip problems. A slight loss of balance results, causing errant shots. Prolotherapy to the loose ligaments helps "tighten up" the athlete's game.

Prolotherapy to the loose ligaments in a person's foot and ankle, along with orthotics, are needed to resolve and athlete's chronic knee complaints.

POST-TREATMENT INSTRUCTIONS

An athlete is generally sore for a couple of days after Prolotherapy. This is because the injections have to go through some muscles to get to the ligaments and tendons. To help the muscle soreness resolve itself sooner, massage therapy and moist heat applied to the area is recommended. Natural products to encourage soft tissue healing, such as bromelain, MSM, or products such as Prolo Max, are recommended.

It is imperative for the athlete not to receive high-velocity manipulation in the areas treated with Prolotherapy, as this could disrupt the growth of tissue. Gentle manipulation techniques, such as myofascial release, strain-counter-strain, or activator gun treatments, are fine. Other modalities that improve circulation and assist the healing from Prolotherapy include acupuncture, Rolfing, electrical stimulation, magnets, infrared heat, and ultrasound.

For those who are more sensitive to pain, medications such as Tylenol and Ultram, which are not anti-inflammatory medications, are permissible. Occasionally a muscle relaxant is needed. It is very important to **avoid** anti-inflammatory medications, as these may decrease the effectiveness of Prolotherapy. Narcotic medications, such as Vicodin, Tylenol with Codeine, and Darvocet should also be avoided because they depress the immune system. Of course, this is not helpful because the immune system is critical for healing after Prolotherapy. Exercising is permitted as soon as the athlete feels ready. Generally, athletes start light workouts two days after Prolotherapy. It is common for an athlete to be doing full workouts by day four after Prolotherapy. The general rule is if a certain activity or exercise hurts significantly, switch to a different one. A small amount of pain is expected while recovering from an injury, but not significant pain. If the athlete receives one Prolotherapy treatment and feels fine, follow-up is still recommended to allow the physician to assess the area for complete healing. If it is still significantly tender, further treatments are needed because the area is still injured. Once the tenderness is gone, the athlete is cured.

It is for this reason that many athletes are saying it is time to get the weakened ligament and tendon tissues repaired. This is why many athletes are curing their sports injuries and enhancing their athletic performance with Prolotherapy. ■

BIBLIOGRAPHY

1. Liu, Y. et al. An in situ study of the influence of a sclerosing solution in rabbit medial collateral ligaments and its junction strength. *Connective Tissue Research*. 1983; 11:95-102.

2. Maynard, JA et al. Morphological and biochemical effects of sodium morrhuate on tendons. *Journal of Orthopaedic Research*. 1985; 3(2):236-248.

3. Hauser, R. *Prolo Your Pain Away!* Oak Park, IL: Beulah Land Press. 1998, p. 123.

4. Scott, W. *Dr. Scott's Knee Book*. New York, NY: Fireside. 1996, p. 36.

5. Woo, S. Injury and repair of the musculoskeletal soft tissues. Park Ridge, IL; *American Academy of Orthopedic Surgeons. 1987*, p. <u>113</u>.

6. Woo, S. Injury and repair of the musculoskeletal soft tissues. Park Ridge, IL; *American Academy of Orthopedic Surgeons*. 1987, p. <u>154</u>.

7. Woo, S. Injury and repair of the musculoskeletal soft tissues. Park Ridge, IL; *American Academy of Orthopedic Surgeons*. 1987, p. <u>155</u>.

8. Woo, S. Injury and repair of the musculoskeletal soft tissues. Park Ridge, IL; *American Academy of Orthopedic Surgeons*. 1987, p. <u>156</u>.

9. Woo, S. Injury and repair of the musculoskeletal soft tissues. Park Ridge, IL; *American Academy of Orthopedic Surgeons*. 1987, p. <u>477</u>.

10. NIH Consensus Statement on Total Hip Replacement. 1994; 12:1-31. Published by the *NIH* in Kensington, Maryland.

11. Cohen, N. Composition and dynamics of articular cartilage; structure, function and maintaining healthy state. *JOSPT.* 1998; 28:203-215.

12. Brukner, P. *Clinical Sports Medicine*. New York City, NY: McGraw-Hill Book Company. 1995, pp. 372-391.

13. Wieder, D. Patellofemoral tracking syndrome. *Rehab. Management.* 1992; October/ November: pp. 115-117.

14. Arroll, B. Patellofemoral pain syndrome. *American Journal of Sports Medicine.* 1997; 25:207-212.

15. Finestone, A. Treatment of overuse patellofemoral pain. Prospective randomized controlled clinical trial in a military setting. *Clinical Orthopaedics.* 1991; 293:208-210.

16. Kannus, P. Effect of intra-articular glycosaminoglycan polysulfate treatment on patellofemoral pain syndrome. A prospective, randomized double-blind trial comparing glycosaminoglycan polysulfate with placebo and quadriceps muscle exercises. *Arthritis and Rheumatism.* 1992; 35:1053-1061.

17. Raatikainen, T. Effect of glycosaminoglycan polysulfate on chondromalacia patellae. A placebo-controlled one-year study. *Acta Orthop Scan.* 1990; 61:43-448.

18. Griffin, L. Orthopedic knowledge update—sports medicine. Rosemont, IL: *American Academy of Orthopedic Surgeons*. 1994, pp. 225.

19. Biomechanics of the musculotendinous unit: relation to athletic performance and injury. *Clinical Sports Medicine.* 1983; 2:71-86.

20. Taunton, J. The role of biomechanics in the epidemiology of injuries. *Sports Medicine.* 1988; 6:107-120.

21. Brukner, P. *Clinical Sports Medicine.* New York City, NY: McGraw-Hill Book Company. 1995.

22. Armstrong, R. *Sports Medicine.* 1986; 3:370-381.

23. Friden, J. *International Journal of Sports Medicine.* 1983; 4:170-176.

24. Friden, J. *European Journal of Applied Physiology.* 1988; 57:360-368.

25. Hikida, R. J. *Neur. Sci.* 1983; 59:185-203.

26. Apple, F. *Clin. Chem. Acta.* 1984; 138:111-118.

27. Schwane, J. *Med. Sci. Sports.* Ex. 1983; 15:51-65.

28. Apple, F. *Journal of Applied Physiology.* 1988; 65:2598-2600.

29. Curwin, S. *Tendonitis: Its Etiology and Treatment.* Lexington: Collamore Press. 1984; pp. 1-67.

30. Hunter-Griffin, L. Overuse injuries. *Clinical Sports Medicine.* 1987; 6:225-466.

31. Perugia, L. *The Tendons: Biology-Pathology-Clinical Aspects.* Milano:Editrice Kurtis. 1986.

32. Pecina, M. *Overuse Injuries of the Musculoskeletal System.* Boca Raton, FL: CRC Press. 1993, pp. 1-26.

33. Ferretti, A. Knee injuries in volleyball. *Sports Medicine.* 1990; 10:132-138.

34. Ferretti, A. Jumper's knee. An epidemiological study of volleyball players. *Physician and .Sportsmedicine.* 1984; 12:97-106.

35. Henry, J. Jumper's knee. *Sport Med. Actual.* 1988; 3:10-13.

36. Janssen, G. Das Patellaspitzensyndrom. *Orthop. Praxis.* 1983; 19:12-15.

37. Pecina, M. Doprinos etiologiji skakackog koljena. *KMV.* 1988; 3:11-14.

38. Kujala, M. Knee injuries in athletes, review of exertion injuries and retrospective study of outpatient sports clinical material. *Sports Medicine.* 1986; 3:195-200.

39. Ferretti, A. Ethiopathogenetic considerations of jumper's knee. *Italian Journal of Sports Trauma.* 1983; 5:101-105.

40. Terry, G. The anatomy of the extensor mechanism. *Clinical Sports Medicine.* 1989; 8:163-179.

41. Pecina, M. *Overuse Injuries of the Musculoskeletal System.* Boca Raton, FL: CRC Press. 1993, pp. 179-193.

42. Ferretti, A. Epidemiology of jumper's knee. *Sports Medicine.* 1986; 3:289-295.

43. Pecina, M. Contribution to the etiological explanation of "basketball knee." *Sports Medicine Actual.* 1988; 3:29-31.

44. Ferretti, A. Jumper's knee. *American Journal of Sports Medicine.* 1983; 11:58-62.

45. Perrugia, L. The Tendons: Biology—Pathology—Clinical Aspects. Milano: Editrice Kurtis. 1986.

46. Colosimo, A. Jumper's knee. *Orthopaedic Review.* 1990; 19:139-149.

47. Basset, F. *AAOS Instructional Course Lectures.* 1976; 25:96-106.

48. Ferretti, A. Jumper's knee. *American Journal of Sports Medicine.* 1983; 11:58-62.

49. Cook, J. A cross-sectional study of 100 athletes with jumper's knee managed conservatively and surgically. *British Journal of Sports Medicine.* 1997; 31:332-336.

50. Popp, J. Recalcitrant patellar tendonitis. *American Journal of Sports Medicine.* 1997; 25:218-222.

51. Kennedy, J. Hawkins, R. Breaststroker's knee. *Physician and Sportsmedicine.* 1974; 2:33-38.

52. Vizsoly, P. Breaststroker's knee. An analysis of epidemiological and biomechanical factors. *American Journal of Sports Medicine.* 1987; 15:63-71.

53. Stulberg, S. Breaststroker's knee: pathology, etiology, and treatment. *American Journal of Sports Medicine.* 1980; 8:164-171.

54. Costill, D. *Handbook of Sports Medicine and Science Swimming.* Oxford: Blackwell Scientific Publications. 1992.

55. Johnson, J. Musculoskeletal injuries in competitive swimmers. *Mayo Clinic Proceedings.* 1987; 62:289-304.

56. Heiser, T. Prophylaxis and management of hamstring muscle injuries in intercollegiate football players. *American Journal of Sports Medicine.* 1984; 12:268-270.

57. Pecina, M. *Overuse Injuries of the Musculoskeletal System.* Boca Raton, FL: CRC Press. 1993, pp. 147-159.

58. La Cava, G. L'enthesite ou maladie des insertions. *Press Med.* 1959; 67:9.

59. Rosenberg, T. Skiing. In Reider, B. (ed.), Sports Medicine— The School-Age Athlete. Philadelphia, PA: W.B. Saunders. 1996, pp. 741-756.

60. Johnson, R. Skier injury trends. Presented at the *Seventh International Symposium on Skiing Trauma and Safety*, France. 1989.

61. Paletta, G. Knee injuries and alpine skiing. *Sports Medicine.* 1994; 6:411-423.

62. Fetto, J., Marshall, J. The natural history and diagnosis of anterior cruciate ligament insufficiency. *Clinical Orthopaedics and Related Research.* 1980; 147:29-38.

63. Anderson, A. Analysis of rehabilitation techniques after anterior crucitate ligament reconstruction. *American Journal of Sports Medicine.* 1989; 17:154-160.

64. Fowler, P. The patient with symptomatic chronic anterior cruciate ligament insufficiency. Results of minimal arthroscopic surgery and rehabilitation. *American Journal of Sports Medicine.* 1987; 15:321-325.

65. McDaniel, J. The untreated anterior cruciate ligament rupture. *Clinical Orthopaedics and Related Research.* 1983; 172:158-163.

66. Boynton, M. Long-term follow-up of the untreated isolated posterior cruciate ligament-deficient knee. *American Journal of Sports Medicine.* 1996; 24:306-310.

67. Keller, P. Nonoperatively treated isolated posterior cruciate ligament injuries. *American Journal of Sports Medicine.* 1993; 21:132-136.

68. Bosch, U. Alterations of glycosaminoglycans during patellar tendon autograft healing after posterior cruciate ligament replacement. *American Journal of Sports Medicine.* 1998; 26:103-108.

69. Richter, M. Primary repair for posterior cruciate ligament injuries—an eight year follow-up of fifty-three patients. *American Journal of Sports Medicine.* 1996; 24:298-305.

70. Dorman, T. *Diagnosis and Injection Techniques in Orthopedic Medicine.* Baltimore, MD: Williams and Wilkins. 1991, pp. 224.

71. Veltri, D. The role of the politeofibular ligament in stability of the human knee. *American Journal of Sports Medicine.* 1996; 24:19-27.

72. Maynard, M. The popliteofibular ligament. *American Journal of Sports Medicine.* 1996; 24:311-316.

CHAPTER 7

Prolo Your Other Knee Pain Away!

Though this is a small book on Prolotherapy, I want to try to include all the knee conditions I can think of in it. The more common conditions (especially affecting athletes) were discussed in the last chapter. This chapter is saved for the "other" knee pains. You know the "others"—the non-athletes. The conditions described in this chapter have mostly to do with the conditions occurring because of a biochemical problem when the person isn't healing well. These injuries are not typically from trauma, but some inherent problem that needs comprehensive natural medicine, in addition to Prolotherapy to fix it. It is like when you ask your wife to do something and she does it. No questions, inquires, just "yes dear." Then you think to yourself "how did that happen?"

THE ARTHRITIDES

There are a lot of people with arthritis. There are two main types of arthritis, degenerative and inflammatory. Degenerative arthritis is also called osteo-arthritis. As explained in this book it generally occurs when there is injury to the joint, specifically the ligaments that stabilize it. Once the ligaments are injured, the muscles have to contract around the joint to protect it. When the muscles can no longer do this the bones around the joint begin to grow, thus the bony spurs indicative of arthritis. This extra bone is the body's attempt to stabilize the joint. Eventually, because of the ligament injuries, the menisci and articular cartilage deteriorate. This is when there is a crunching or grating sound in the joint. Eventually the joint wears down until there is "bone on bone." Prolotherapy is a great treatment for degenerative arthritis because it helps repair the ligament injury which started the arthritic process in the first place.

The other main type of arthritis is called inflammatory arthritis. The most common inflammatory arthritis is rheumatoid arthritis. Other types of inflammatory arthritis are psoriatic arthritis, Lyme Disease, lupus, gouty arthritis, and chondrocalcinosis or pseudogout. The characteristic of inflammatory arthritides are that they cause swelling and stiffness in the joint. In rheumatoid arthritis the swelling typically occurs symmetrically and in the hands. All of the various arthritides can affect all the joints including the knee joint.

The difference between degenerative and inflammatory arthritis is the fact that Prolotherapy gets at the root cause of the condition, ligament weakness or laxity. In regard to inflammatory arthritis, Prolotherapy often gets at the root cause of the pain but not the underlying condition. So when faced with a patient who has an inflammatory arthritide, Prolotherapy plus comprehensive natural medicine is warranted.

The natural medicine approach to conditions such as Lyme Disease, rheumatoid arthritis, and lupus include doing diagnostic testing for food allergies, infections, and various nutritional factors. If an infection is found this is treated with appropriate antibiotics or antifungal medications. Foods for which there are allergies are eliminated from the diet. Nutritional factors are treated by changes in diet and vitamin and herbal supplementation. *(See Appendix G on nutritional supplements.)* Because inflammatory arthritis can damage the joints, Prolotherapy is used to help stimulate the repair of the joints. Prolotherapy is helpful to relieve the pain of inflammatory arthritis, but if not combined with a comprehensive natural medicine approach, the pain will just recur.

A CASE OF CHONDROCALCINOSIS

Born January 19, 1971, his name is Michael Myung Soo.* His resume in Tae Kwon Do reads as follows:

1997　U.S. Open; U.S. Olympic Training Center • Silver—Men's Feather

1996　World University Games; St. Petersburg, Russia • Silver—Men's Feather, U.S. Team Trials; U.S. Olympic Training Center • Bronze—Men's Feather, World University Team Trials • Gold—Men's Feather

1995　U.S. Collegiate Nationals; New York, NY • Gold—Men's Feather

1993　Korean American Sports Festival; Chicago, Illinois • Gold—Men's Feather, U.S. Collegiate Nationals; Tibadaux, LA • Gold—Men's Feather

Some of his other accomplishments include 10-time Washington State Champion (1985-1995), Junior Olympic Champion (Gold—139 pound class—1987), and host of other national and international championships. He was one of 12 Tae Kwon Do athletes nationwide selected for the United States Olympic Training Center Resident Athlete Program as he trained for the Olympic Games in Sydney, Australia, in 2000.

In looking at Michael's accomplishments one thing stands out—besides the fact that this guy is awesome. What happened in 1994? He had an injury. For six months, he tried everything to recoup a very painful, weak knee. He was unable to kick and compete effectively for six months.

He was getting nowhere with heat, ice, ibuprofen, exercise and physiotherapy, so he went to see Richard Koch, D.O., for Prolotherapy. "I was thinking my career and dreams were over. I really wanted to compete in the Olympics. That was where I was heading but, because of my knee, I was no longer able to lunge and kick like I needed. My performances in tournaments were suffering greatly. In 1994, I wasn't doing too well emotionally, either." Dr. Koch performed Prolotherapy once per month for four months on Michael's medial collateral ligament, which was torn. Some intra-articular (inside) knee injections were given because he had evidence of chondrocalcinosis throughout the knee.

Chondrocalcinosis is a disease characterized by calcified deposits, free from urate and consisting of calcium pyrophosphate crystals, in synovial fluid,

---

* *Name has been changed to protect patient's privacy.*

articular cartilage, and adjacent soft tissue. It causes various forms of arthritis commonly characterized by gout-like attacks of pain, swelling of the involved joints, and radiologic evidence of calcification in articular cartilage. This condition is also know as pseudogout. "Even after the first two sessions of Prolotherapy, I felt a difference. I started jogging again. I could definitely tell my knee was getting stronger. By the fourth series I was completely well. I couldn't wait to start competing again. Since my knee injury was healed back in 1994, I have won just about every tournament I have entered. I am sure Prolotherapy is the way to go when an athlete has a sports injury. It was the only treatment that worked for me." Yes, Michael, you are not alone. For many athletes, Prolotherapy is the only treatment that is doing the work for them, too!

ELDERLY KNEE PAIN

"My knee pain is slowing me down, can you fix it?!" Mr. Walgreen was always to the point. The son of the founder of Walgreen's pharmacy and chairman of the board of Walgreens during his prime, was 94 years old when he said those words to me. He and his wife were still traveling around the world. They both received Prolotherapy. I saw him many years later because he had unremitted shoulder pain. He knew where to turn...Prolotherapy.

The reason why I have this section is that pain is no respecter of person, age, or sex. All people whether they are in their 90s or a young child deserve the chance to be pain free. Regular pains can occur in children, teenagers, and of course the elderly. The same process as described in this book is done for all with generally the same result, no pain.

KNEE INJURIES

Knee injury and pain is also quite common in the older athlete. Again, the hiker, square dancer, tennis player, basketball player, and bicyclist frequently find that knee pain has increased after performing their favorite sport. Pain can be due to osteoarthritis of the knee joint, arthritis behind the patella (kneecap), sprain of the ligaments on the inner and outer part of the knee (medial and lateral collateral ligaments), and weakness of ligaments inside the knee (anterior and posterior cruciate ligaments). *(See Figure 7-1.)* Generally all that is needed is a good history and physical examination to

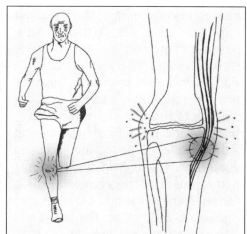

Figure 7-1: Athletic Knee Injury in the Older Athlete
Decreased joint space and "bone spurs" are two of the signs of degenerative joint disease, which is more prevalent in the older athlete. Prolotherapy can prevent this.

determine exactly which component of the knee is injured.

There are specific tests on the knee in order to determine the strength of the ligaments. These tests are relatively painless and involve pulling the lower leg forward or backward (anterior or posterior drawer test), pressure on the inner or outer lower leg to determine weakness of the side ligaments (valgus and varus stress test), and listening for crepitus in the joints. *(See Figure 7-2.)* Occasionally x-rays or MRIs are ordered, usually to confirm a diagnosis.

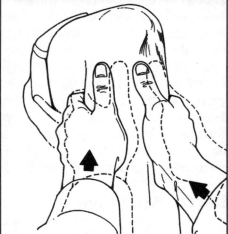

Figure 7-2: Anterior Drawer Test of the Knee
If the knee moves with this test, weakness of the anterior cruciate ligament is the cause.

Once the diagnosis has been made, generally, Prolotherapy is indicated because almost all knee pain is soft tissue in origin. Prolotherapy can be quite useful in strengthening the medial and lateral collateral ligaments of the knee. It will eliminate pain on the inner and outer aspect of the knee. Tightening the ligaments surrounding the knee, along with injection of a proliferant solution into the joint of the knee, can frequently help osteoarthritis pain. Injection of proliferant into the knee helps to tighten the joint capsule. In addition, rehabilitation may also be recommended and usually includes exercises to strengthen the muscle surrounding the knee, flexibility training of the muscles of the leg and back, and physiotherapies to help tender points in the muscles (trigger points). As a side note, one of the best exercises that improves coordination, flexibility, and proprioception, as well as muscle strength, is jump roping. **Real men jump rope!** *(See Figure 7-3.)*

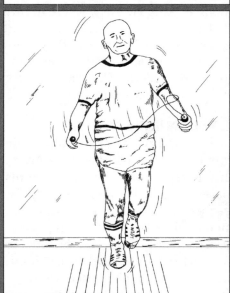

Figure 7-3: Real "Older" Men Jump Rope
A simple exercise like jumping rope helps improve coordination, flexibility, proprioception, as well as muscle strength.

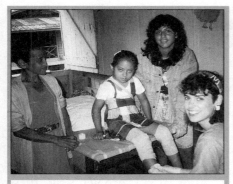

Figure 7-4:
Marion assists Joanna, a Down's Syndrome patient in Honduras.

LIGAMENT LAXITY: AN OVERLOOKED PROBLEM IN CHILDREN

"Joanna's knees keep dislocating," said her frantic mother. Joanna was four years old with Down's Syndrome. She received Prolotherapy to the knees. She went through the treatment without a twinge. *(See Figure 7-4)* She was great. The results were great too!

Joint laxity, or the looseness of a joint, can have a major impact on not only an athlete's ability to excel in a sport, but also the likelihood of injury. A good example of this is gymnastics. The greater the joint laxity in the child, the more likely that child will be able to do all of the required contortion movements in gymnastics. Many people derive an added advantage in their pursuit of athletics, acrobatics, and ballet dancing, where greater flexibility is an asset.[1] For the young tennis player, the greater the laxity in the shoulder joint, the more power that can be obtained in the serve. Joint laxity can have tremendous benefits to the athlete, but it is a double-edged sword. The greater the joint laxity, the more likely the joint is going to suffer a sports-related injury. As it turns out, a person generally has the greatest flexibility as a child.[2] An often overlooked fact in sports medicine in children is that they have the most mobile joints on the planet! Their joints are already stretched. It does not take much more to get their joints pathologically hypermobile (injured).

Joint laxity is primarily a function of the ligaments that connect the bones together. The stronger the ligaments, the more stable the joint. The more lax the ligaments, the looser the joint and the more prone to injury. Generalized joint hypermobility due to ligamentous laxity occurs in about five percent of the population.[3] Hypermobile joints are exhibited by being able to do things, such as bending the elbow or knee past the neutral position; touching the floor with the palm while bending at the waist; doing the splits; and touching the thumb to the forearm. Usually these people are always entertaining their friends with these skills. Unfortunately, repeatedly performing these acts usually leads to injury down the road. In subtler cases, this condition can only be determined by a physical examination—one of the reasons it is not diagnosed by most physicians. Most physicians are not trained to adequately examine a patient for joint mobility and ligament laxity. Doctors who perform Prolotherapy routinely examine ligaments and look for joint laxity because the treatment of choice for hypermobility syndrome or a loose joint is Prolotherapy. It is only Prolotherapy that can strengthen the joint capsule and ligaments to keep an athlete's joints stable enough to allow the athletes to excel in their respective sports.

COMMON SITES FOR OVERUSE and APOPHYSIS INJURIES

SITE	ASSOCIATED SPORTS	DISEASE NAME
Tibia tubercle	Jumping, sprinting, skiing, soccer	Osgood-Schlatter disease
Patella (inferior pole)	Soccer, rugby, jumping sprinting, skiing	Sinding-Larsen-Johansson syndrome
Calcaneous	Running, aerobics, soccer	Sever's disease
Navicular	Sprinting, running, aerobics	Kohler's disease
Olecranon	Throwing, tennis, gymnastics, wt. lifting	Little League elbow
Lunate	Tennis, throwing, martial arts	Keinbock's disease
2nd Metatarsal head	Dancing, kicking sports	Freiberg's disease

Adapted from D. F. Gerrard, Overuse injury and growing bones. British Journal of Sports Medicine © 1993; 27: 14-18

Figure 7-5: Common Sites for Overuse Apophysis Injuries
Instead of rest, young athletes need strengthening of the soft tissues and joints to heal the above injuries. The best way to do that is Prolotherapy.

This topic has been studied to see if athletic injuries could be predicted. As it turns out, excessive joint laxity is the main risk factor for recurrent ligamentous injury.[4] Pathologic joint laxity, especially about the knee and shoulder, are the main risk factors for young athletes for recurrent problems in these areas.[5-7] If the joint laxity is not addressed, joint dislocations occur with the end result being osteoarthritis.[8,9] Every time a young athlete's joint dislocates, their chance of developing degenerative osteoarthritis as an adult increases. For this reason, any athlete sustaining a joint dislocation is encouraged to get an evaluation by a Prolotherapist to make sure that the joint laxity has resolved. Prolotherapy is the treatment of choice for any athlete, regardless of age, for recurrent joint dislocations. The ligament strength in children and young athletes has been overlooked as one of the associated factors regarding children developing one of the more common apophysitis. *(See Figure 7-5.)*

Treatment of apophyseal injury should start by looking at the ligament laxity in the young athlete, not in how can we stop the athlete's sports development by limiting innings pitched or soccer kicks, etc. Ligament laxity is almost always found with athletic injuries in the young. They are more prone to getting it because of the normal joint laxity found in them. Prolotherapy, to the ligament laxity, makes the joint stronger and heals not only the ligament laxity, but also the apophyseal injury. In this way the athlete can return to athletics quicker, but also in stronger form. Because the underlying cause of the apophysitis has been treated, the likelihood of recurrence is much less. *(See Figure 7-6.)*

OSGOOD-SCHLATTER DISEASE: APOPHYSITIS OF THE KNEE

Chronic knee pain may develop in young athletes, especially teenagers, and is often due to Osgood-Schlatter Disease, a condition whereby the tibial tubercle becomes painful where the patellar tendon attaches to the tibia. Pain occurs because there is tendon weakness at the same area of the tibia that is growing. *(See Figure 7-7.)* The pain is exacerbated by physical activity, especially running and jumping, and often limits participation in sports, resulting in the young athlete's physicians recommending cessation of playing sports. Needless to say, this advice is not popular. A better treatment is to strengthen the fibro-osseous junction of the patellar tendon onto the tibial tubercle, eliminating the problem. In a small study published in 1993, Prolotherapy was 83 percent effective in eliminating the pain of Osgood-Schlatter Disease.[10] In this study only one to two treatments were needed to resolve the problem.

WOMEN ARE MUCH LOOSER THAN MEN— AND WE'RE NOT TALKING ABOUT MORALS!

Walk into any chronic pain clinic and who do you see? You see women. Caring Medical and Rehabilitation Services in Oak Park is no different. About three out of every four patients coming for Prolotherapy are woman. Why? Aren't the guys the ones getting all banged up playing basketball, football, and doing the physical work around the house? (Yeah, right!) Why are the women getting most of the arthritis and needing the majority of the artificial joint replacements? It is easy to explain when you take into account the hormone factor.

The dominant hormone in males is testosterone. Testosterone is very anabolic, which means that it stimulates the growth or repair of tissues. Men have about 10 times

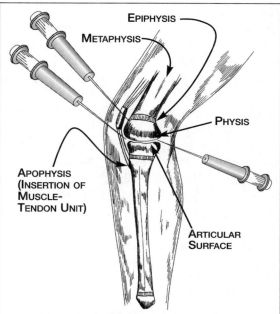

Figure 7-6: Prolotherapy and the Young Athlete's Knee
Prolotherapy to the growth plate area (epiphysis), ligament and tendon attachments (apophysis), or ligament-bone interfaces (fibro-osseous junction) will assist in actually strengthening and repairing the areas.

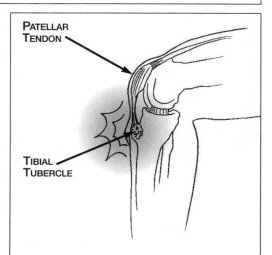

Figure 7-7: Osgood-Schlatter Disease
Patellar tendon weakness leads to tibial tuberal swelling characteristic of Osgood-Schlatter Disease.

the amount of testosterone as women. This is why they have a sex drive that is about 10 times as strong as women do. It is also the reason why, on average, men are 33 percent stronger than women.[11] Males are stronger because of their increased muscle mass due to testosterone. When males perform strength training, they develop increased strength and increased muscle size due to hypertrophy of the muscles. This hypertrophy is due to the effect of testosterone. Females performing strength training gain increased strength with relatively less muscle hypertrophy. This is because females have significantly less testosterone. If a woman shows up at the Olympics looking like a man, the other athletes will accuse her of using anabolic hormones like testosterone. The complaint is justified. When a woman does weight strength training, she will get stronger, but she cannot turn herself into a body shaped like a man because the hormones are just not there.

Recent epidemiological studies have recognized a significantly higher anterior cruciate ligament (ACL) injury rate in female athletes as compared with male athletes in sports such as basketball, handball, gymnastics, and soccer.[12-15] Although various causes of this phenomenon have been postulated, including differences in ligament or muscle strength, conditioning, endurance, anatomy, and training techniques, the most plausible appears to be the hormone factor.[16] Unique to the female athlete is her exposure to a constantly changing hormonal milieu throughout her reproductive years. For most of her life, the female athlete is exposed to rhythmic variation in either endogenous hormones during a regular menstrual cycle or exogenous hormones via oral contraceptives.

It has been only recently that it was discovered that there are **estrogen receptors** on the fibro-blasts of the human ACL, suggesting that female sex hormones may have an effect on the structure and composition of this ligament. Dr. Stephen Liu and associates, at the UCLA School of Medicine, made this discovery and went the next step to find out exactly how estrogen affects ligament growth. They investigated the effects of 17B-estradiol on the cellular proliferation and collagen synthesis of fibroblasts derived from the rabbit anterior cruciate ligament. Measuring 3H-thymidine and 14C-hydroxyproline incorporation assessed fibroblast proliferation and collagen synthesis, respectively. They found that collagen synthesis was significantly reduced with increasing local estradiol concentration. Declining collagen synthesis was first noted at a 17B-estradiol concentration of 0.025 ng/ml. Within physiologic levels of estrogen (0.025 to 0.25 ng/ml), collagen synthesis was reduced by more than 40 percent of control, and at pharmacological levels of 2.5 and 25 ng/ml, as typically occurs in female athletes taking birth control pills or estrogen replacement therapy, by more than 50 percent of control. A significant reduction of fibroblast proliferation was also observed with increasing estradiol concentrations. *(See Figure 7-8.)*

These results are startling. They should make every female athlete shake in her sneakers. **Estrogen, the female hormone, dramatically inhibits fibroblasts.**

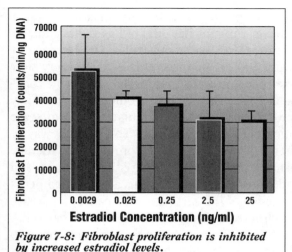

Figure 7-8: Fibroblast proliferation is inhibited by increased estradiol levels.

Adapted from American Journal of Sports Medicine, Vol. 25, P. 707, ©1998

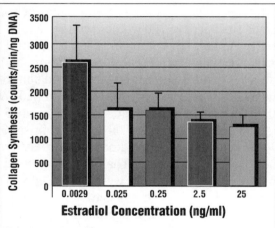

Figure 7-9: Collagen Synthesis is inhibited by Increased Estradiol Levels.

Adapted from American Journal of Sports Medicine, Vol. 25, P. 707, ©1998

These fibroblasts are what make the collagen that makes up the ligaments and tendons, which are injured during sports. Estrogen was shown in the above study to inhibit the fibroblastic growth and thus collagen formation in a dose-dependent manner. *(See Figure 7-9.)* The more estrogen a woman has, the more inhibition will occur. This has direct effects for all women taking birth control pills. Birth control pills have pharmacological levels of estrogen, which are far in excess of a woman's normal production. The simplest way for a female athlete, who is on artificial estrogen, to overcome sports injuries, is to stop taking them. Inevitably, women are placed on birth control pills because of menstrual irregularities, which are easily treated with natural medicine techniques including diet manipulation and nutritional supplements.

Because of the double whammy of estrogen and relaxin, (another hormone more prominent in women) women have increased ligamentous laxity and flexibility compared to their male counterparts.[17, 18, 19] This excessive laxity is the reason that there is an increased incidence of patellar subluxations and ligament sprains seen in female athletes.[20, 21] This laxity is especially present during pregnancy when the risk of ankle sprains and ligamentous injuries is highest.[22] If this was not bad enough, articular cartilage has estrogen receptors located on it. Like ligamentous tissue, estrogen has a direct negative effect on cartilage growth and repair.[23]

The net effect of all of this is that the joints of females, even females who have no pain whatsoever, are not normal. They cannot possibly be normal because of all the negative effects of estrogen as the prime instigator and relaxin as a lessor instigator. Remember that the turnover time (or half-life) of ligaments and cartilage is about one to two years. This means that about half of the cartilage or ligaments is regenerated about every 300 to 700 days. This is a very, very slow rate. Fibroblastic cells, which make collagen, and chondrocytes that make cartilage tissue, are stable cells in the fact that they do not proliferate easily. They need to be stimulated to proliferate. Injury to tissue stimulates them to some degree, but exercise does not noticeably change this rate. The primary way to stimulate the fibroblasts and chondrocytes is by direct proliferative therapy (Prolotherapy). Prolotherapy injections are given right where the fibroblasts and chondrocytes are located—at the fibro-osseous junction. This is where ligaments attach to bone or directly on the outside of the cartilage. This causes a massive stimulation of fibroblastic and chondrocyte growth, with the net effect being ligament and cartilage growth. It is this treatment that offers the only hope to women to not only get rid of their chronic pain, but also cure their sports injuries. As you will see, even women without any pain have weak joints.

Dr. Lanny Johnson and associates from the Department of Surgery, College of Human Medicine, Michigan State University, in East Lansing, published a landmark study in 1998. They analyzed the knees of 100 women who were totally asymptomatic of any problems in their knees. The volunteers completed a uniform comprehensive medical history questionnaire, physical examination, and plain film radiographs. The study showed that **95 percent** of women had abnormal findings in their knees.[19] The women were the average age of 47 and had an average lifetime-sports hours of 6,090. The data is startling: Q-angle degrees: 15; patellofemoral crepitus (crunching): 94 percent; unaware of their crepitus: 89 percent; lateral patellar mobility: 99 percent; and excessive knee hyperextension (evidence of significant knee ligament laxity): 42 percent. The findings on x-ray were equally impressive. The x-rays on these asymptomatic women showed scalloping sclerosis, osteophytes, bone spurs, and every other degenerative change. The activity level of these women, for the most part, was moderate in 66 and vigorous in 21 of the participants. Remember, this study used a strict criterion that the women had to have been totally asymptomatic in their knees for a lifetime. Women need to learn about natural ways to balance their hormones and the best method of curing the associated ligament laxity-Prolotherapy.

ARE YOU CATABOLIC OR ANABOLIC?

Perhaps one of the most important questions people with pain—especially women—could ask themselves is this one: are you catabolic or anabolic? According to *Merriam Webster's Collegiate Dictionary, 10th Edition*, catabolism refers to the "destructive metabolism involving the release of energy and resulting in the breakdown of complex materials within the organism, whereas anabolism refers to the constructive part of metabolism concerned with macromolecular synthesis." In common language, this means that a catabolic process

FIGURE 7-10	CATABOLIC	ANABOLIC
Estradiol Levels	*High*	*Low*
Estriol Levels	*Low*	*High*
Progesterone Levels	*Low*	*High*
DHEA Levels	*Low*	*High*
Growth Hormone Levels	*Low*	*High*
Testosterone Levels	*Low*	*High*
Aging Effects	*Advanced*	*Diminished*
Arthritis Risk	*High*	*Low*
Connective Tissue Healing	*Poor*	*Excellent*
Recovery After Workouts	*Poor*	*Excellent*
Ability to Train Intensely	*Poor*	*Excellent*
Likelihood of Injury	*High*	*Low*
Healing Capacity	*Poor*	*High*

Figure 7-10: Catabolic versus Anabolic Profiles

A person who is anabolic has a much greater chance of having their injuries heal more completely than a catabolic person.

involves the breakdown of materials, whereas an anabolic process involves the building up or synthesis of the materials. It is imperative that the athlete desiring to excel in his/her sports, by getting stronger and faster, maintain an anabolic profile. Refer to *Figure 7-10* to see how important anabolism is to enhancing athletic performance. The athlete will maintain the ability to train hard, repair muscles, ligaments and tendons that are exercised, and heal injuries if they occur. If the athlete becomes catabolic, however, workouts will become more difficult, as evidenced by lingering soreness and chronic sports injuries will become inevitable.

Certain testing procedures can be done in order to document an athlete's state of anabolism or catabolism. The first areas that are usually checked are the hormones, including estradiol, progesterone, cortisol, DHEA, testosterone, and Growth Hormone. Estradiol stimulates catabolism, whereas DHEA, testosterone, progesterone, and Growth Hormone are anabolic. Abnormal (too low or too high) Cortisol levels promote catabolism. If cortisol levels are too low, supplementation with natural Cortisol is warranted.

Since catabolism means breakdown of materials, measuring the level of breakdown products of certain substances will determine the amount of catabolism for that particular substance. As previously discussed, the breakdown product of collagen is hydroxyproline. This can be measured in the blood and the urine to assess the state of catabolism of collagen in the active patient. For the person found to be in a catabolic state, natural hormone replacement and dietary changes can be made. After a couple months, the tests can repeated to make sure the person's physiology is now anabolic.

FIBROMYALGIA—ANOTHER CONSEQUENCE OF HIGH ESTRADIOL

Whiplash injuries, back strains, ankle sprains, loose joints, fibromyalgia, and sports injuries all have weakness or deficiency in the soft tissues of the body as their root cause. Fibromyalgia is a condition where the weakness or deficiency in the soft tissues is *everywhere*. The condition effects many more women than men, mainly because of the high estradiol in women. As discussed previously, estradiol inhibits fibroblastic proliferation, thus the propensity for women to suffer from chronic pain. If many areas of the body become effected, the muscles throughout the body get characteristic trigger (tender) points. It is then the person gets labeled with the diagnosis of fibromyalgia.

To make the diagnosis of Fibromyalgia, one of the cardinal features is tenderness over specific points on the body. The diagnosis is made when at least 11 of the 18 points are tender. The unilateral sites are the occiput (insertion of the suboccipital muscles), inter-transverse ligaments C5-C7, trapezius muscle, origin of the supraspinatous muscle, second costochondral junction (ligament), lateral epicondyle (wrist extensor muscle insertions), gluteal area (gluteus maximus muscle), greater trochanter (gluteus medius muscle insertion), and the medial fat pad of the knee (medial collateral ligament). In essence, 14 of the 18 points are located where either a ligament, tendon, or muscle inserts and the remaining four are in the middle of a particular muscle. Prolotherapy grows ligament, tendon, and muscle tissue where they attach to the bone, thus eliminating trigger points and the pain of Fibromyalgia.

Whether a patient has been given the label of Fibromyalgia, Myofascial Pain Syndrome, or post-surgical pain syndrome, the hallmark feature typically is very sensitive trigger point areas. The person often feels a knot in the muscle in that area. These areas are called "trigger points" because they trigger a person's pain if compressed and palpated and cause the positive "jump sign." Trigger points also refer pain to a distal site that becomes painful. In a study published in 1994, K. Dean Reeves, M.D., showed that even in people with severe Fibromyalgia, Prolotherapy caused a reduction in pain levels and increased functional abilities in more than 75 percent of patients.[24] In 38 percent of the patients, Prolotherapy was the only effective treatment they ever received. An additional 25 percent said that Prolotherapy was much more effective than any previous treatment. The study showed that overall, 90 percent of the severe Fibromyalgia patients benefitted from the Prolotherapy injections.

What does fibromyalgia have to do with knee pain? Not much, but this is the unusual pain chapter, so everything is free game. Fibromyalgia does cause significant knee pain by the pes anserine area. The pain of fibromyalgia can be tremendously helped by Prolotherapy but the underlying physiology associated with the condition must also be treated through comprehensive natural medicine to truly rid the person of their body pain. This treatment can incorporate natural anabolic hormone replacement, including growth hormone, testosterone, or DHEA. Appropriate nutritional supplements that help heal soft tissues are also typically recommended. *(See Appendix G.)*

STRESS FRACTURES

Since we are talking about healing, one of the more common causes of pain coming from non-healing conditions—especially in female athletes—are stress fractures. These are a rare cause of knee pain but a common cause of lower leg pain. Stress fractures most commonly occur in the lower extremities, but also occur in non-weight-bearing bones, including the ribs, upper extremities, and the pelvis. The most common sites are the tibia, metatarsals, and fibula. A recent study demonstrated a high incidence of tarsal navicular stress fractures, which may be the most common site in certain groups such as sprinters and hurdlers. Sports associated with specific stress fractures include rowing and golf (ribs), baseball pitching (humerus), and gymnastics (spine) and are shown in *Figure 7-11.*[25]

Recent studies have shown that the incidence of stress fractures in athletes is higher than previously thought. As you can see from *Figure 7-11*, the most frequent sport associated with stress fractures is running. One prospective study of 95 track and field athletes showed an annual incidence of approximately 20 percent.[26]

The mainstay traditional treatment for stress fractures is rest. The theory behind this is that the bone is breaking down faster than it can be built up (because of the running), therefore rest is needed. A better approach is to view stress fractures as a connective tissue deficiency of the bone and to determine why that exact area is weakened. *(See Figure 7-12.)*

FIGURE 7-11: STRESS FRACTURE SITES ASSOCIATED WITH SPECIFIC SPORTS AND ACTIVITIES

SITE	SPORT OR ACTIVITY
Coracoid Process of Scapula	Trapshooting
Scapula	Running with hand-held weights, Rowing
Humerus	Throwing, Racket Sports
Olecranon	Throwing, Pitching, Javelin
Ulna	Racket Sports (especially Tennis), Gymnastics, Volleyball, Swimming, Softball, Wheelchair Sports, Javelin
Ribs (first)	Throwing, Pitching
Ribs (other)	Rowing, Kayaking
Pars Interarticularis	Gymnastics, Ballet, Cricket, Volleyball, Springboard Diving
Pubic Ramus	Distance Running, Ballet, Swimming
Femur (neck)	Distance Running, Jumping, Ballet
Femure (shaft)	Distance Running
Patella	Running, Hurdling
Tibia (shaft)	Running, Ballet
Fibula	Running, Aerobics, Racewalking, Ballet
Medial Malleolus	Basketball, Running
Calcaneus	Long-Distance Marching, Running
Talus	Pole Vaulting
Navicular	Sprinting, Middle-Distance Running, Hurdling, Long Jumping, Triple Jumping, Football (Australian Rules)
Metatarsal (general)	Running, Ballet, Marching
Metatarsal (fifth)	Tennis, Ballet
Sesamoid Bones of Foot	Running, Ballet, Basketball, Skating

Adapted from Brukner PD, Khan KM, Clinical Sports Medicine, Sydney, McGraw-Hill Book Co, ©1993, p. 17.

Women reportedly have a higher rate of stress fractures than men.[25] It has been found that many female runners who sustain stress fractures have a significantly later age of menarche (onset of menstruation), less menses per year, lower bone mineral density at the spine, and less lower-rib lean mass.[27-30] In addition, female distance runners are known to have a high incidence of eating disorders, which itself may lead to amenorrhea or nutritional deficiencies.[31] In one prospective study, females with lower bone density, history of menstrual disturbance, less lean mass in the lower limbs, a discrepancy in leg length, and who consume a very low fat diet were at a significant risk for stress fractures. No significant risk factors were identified in men; however, there was a strong trend toward low bone density,[32] signifying that stress fractures are a connective tissue deficiency problem in both men and women since the mineral content of the bone was decreased. It is generally accepted, even in traditional medicine circles, that low mineral content in bone is often due to a deficiency in anabolic hormone production. *Figure 7-13* shows the significant drop in hormone production as women age. The same occurs for a man, just at slower rates. Part of healing stress fractures, even in young athletes, is making sure the endocrine (hormonal) system is working properly. This is part of the connective tissue proliferation (collagen-rebuilding) program at our office in Oak Park, Illinois.

The best approach to curing

TIBIA OR FIBULA STRESS FRACTURE

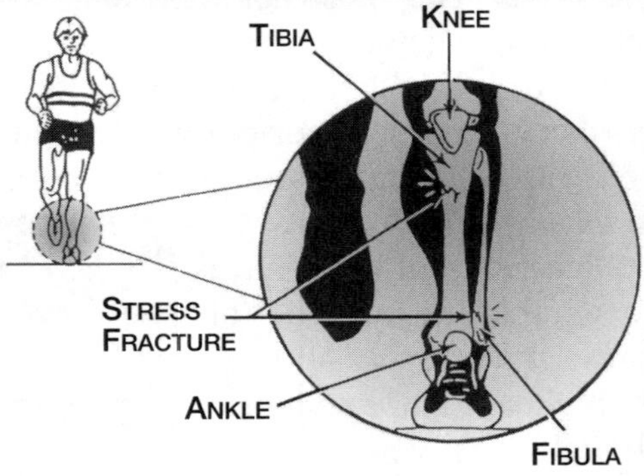

Figure 7-12: Tibia or Fibula Stress Fracture
Stress fractures are best thought of as a weakness or connective tissue deficiency of the bone. Correcting the reason for the deficiency is a much better approach than weakening the athlete with rest and NSAIDs.

Used by permission of Gary N. Guten, M.D., Play Healthy, Stay Healthy, Your Guide to Managing and Treating 40 Common Sports Injuries, Champaign, IL, Leisure Press (A Division of Human Kinetics) © 1991, p. 149.

stress fractures is not to totally eliminate an athlete's training. Imagine how long it took the runner to work up to 35 miles per week. All of the sprint training and weight lifting he/she did day after day all goes out the window because of one injury. This does not have to be the case! All that needs to be done is to treat the exact area of the stress fracture with Prolotherapy. Prolotherapy will cause a strengthening of the fibro-osseous (ligament-bone) junction in the area of the stress fracture. Thus the bone covering (periosteum) is strengthened, as well as the ligamentous and tendon/muscular attachments to the area. To increase circulation to the area, Neural Therapy injections are given around the site of the stress fractures. Generally the athlete feels much better after two or three sessions, given one week apart. To strengthen the inside of the bone, nutritional and/or hormonal supplementation may be needed and should definitely be addressed.*

THE ROLE OF HORMONES IN STRESS FRACTURES

Females are fortunate because they have a monthly guide to assess their nutritional status, the menstrual cycle. A women who has a normal menstrual cycle without PMS or cramping, is generally hormonally and nutritional healthy. Unfortunately, most female athletes who walk through the doors of Caring Medical are not typically in good hormonal or nutritional shape. Many of them are already on oral contraceptive pills (birth control pills) to regulate

---

* *Some of the bone- and connective tissue-building nutriceuticals in our office are Pro Collagen, Skin & Nails, Prolo Max, and RR-6—just to name a few. Call 1-877-RX-BEULAH or visit us on-line at www.benuts.com, for more information.*

BLOOD PRODUCTION RATES OF STEROIDS IN FEMALES

	Reproduction Age	Post-Menopausal
Androstenedione	2-3 mg/day	0.5-1.0 mg/day
Dehydroepiandrosterone	6-8 mg/day	1.5-4.0 mg/day
DHEA-Sulfate	8-16 mg/day	4.9 mg/day
Testosterone	0.2-0.25 mg/day	0.5-1.0 mg/day
Estrogen	0.350 mg/day	0.45 mg/day

Figure 7-13: Blood Production Rates of Steroids in Females
Notice that after menopause, estrogen levels actually increase, yet this is what is prescribed to most women by conventional doctors. Natural medicine physicians put middle-aged women and men on complete natural hormone regimens. This may include DHEA, testosterone, progesterone, and even Growth Hormone. Stress fractures are just one of many conditions that athletes get that have as its root cause connective tissue deficiency from low anabolic hormone levels.

Adapted from A. Lewin, Townsend Letter for Doctors and Patients, © 1996, p. 161-162.

their cycles. This is not a wise move for many reasons. First and foremost, regulating a woman's cycle is extremely easy using dietary and nutritional supplementation. Second, taking birth control pills to cover up the underlying menstrual problem is as bad as taking anti-inflammatory medications to cover up pain. Menstrual irregularities indicate that something in the patient's nutritional and/or hormonal milieu is wrong. Athletes are notorious for covering up problems. Female athletes, you know better than that. Do not cover up menstrual problems by popping birth control pills.

If you are taking birth control pills for birth control's sake, stop that too. If you give a guy his cake and allow him to eat it too, the likelihood of that guy being your long-time mate is dramatically diminished. What a guy wants is a prim and proper gal. Just ask them. Ross used to give talks to high school students on the topic of AIDS prevention. He always asked the students if they wanted to marry virgins. Without fail the majority of students, male and female, would raise their hands. We waited, and trust us, it was worth the wait.

Lastly, oral contraceptive pills have side effects including increasing a woman's risk for stroke and blood clot formation. More importantly, taking birth control pills covers up what is really going on with the woman's menstrual cycle. For this reason the menstrual cycle cannot be used as a marker of the woman's overall health. This book is about solving problems. If the female athlete truly desires to excel in her sport, then the birth control pill must be eliminated.

Often when female athletes are undergoing Metabolic Typing, we find that the fat content in their blood is dangerously low or that they require more fat in their diets than they are currently eating. This is a key factor in helping them heal better. Supplementing with cod liver oil and flaxseed oil, as well as increasing the amounts of fresh fish, nuts, and seeds in the diet, corrects the essential fatty acid deficiency in their bodies. Once this occurs, the hormones become more balanced and the menstrual cycle irregularities cease in many cases. Additional nutritional supplements are given in some cases to help the athlete heal the stress fractures, which may include things like MSM, bromelain, gotu kola, calcium, vitamin D, and other stimulants to connective tissue growth.

SUMMARY

Chronic pain has a cause. The cause involves weakness in a soft tissue structure. Prolotherapy cures pain by strengthening the structure causing the pain. Inflammatory arthritides, apophysitis, degenerative joint disease, ligament laxity, fibromyalgia, and most other causes of knee pain in both young and old, male and female have soft tissue weakness or deficiency as their root cause of the pain. Prolotherapy is successful in treating the pain of these conditions because it stimulates the body to repair the painful structures. To keep the pain away, the underlying cause of these conditions must be treated. In females this can be due to the high estradiol levels in their system. By using comprehensive natural medicine, in addition to Prolotherapy, people with other knee pain can keep their pain away! ■

BIBLIOGRAPHY

1. Grahame, R. Clinical manifestations of the joint hypermobility syndrome. *Reumatologia* (USSR). 1986; 2:20-24.

2. Grahame, R. The hypermobility syndrome. *Annals of Rheumatic Diseases*. 1990; 49:190-200.

3. McCarty, D. *Arthritis and Allied Conditions*. Twelfth Edition. Lea and Febiger, 1993.

4. Lysens, R. The predictability of sports injuries. *Sports Medicine*. 1984; 1:6-10.

5. Goldberg, B. Pre-participation sports assessment—an objective evaluation. *Pediatrics*. 1980; 66:736-745.

6. Nicholas, J. Risk factors, sports medicine and the orthopedic system: an overview. *Sports Medicine*. 1976; 3:243-259.

7. Keller, C. The medical aspects of soccer injury epidemiology. *American Journal of Sports Medicine*. 1987; 15:230-237.

8. Crosby, E. Recurrent dislocation of the patella. Relation of treatment to osteoarthritis. *Journal of Bone and Joint Surgery*. 1976; 58:9-13.

9. Hughstone, J. Subluxation of the patella. *Journal of Bone and Joint Surgery*. 1968; 50:1003-1026.

10. Kidd, R. Recent developments in the understanding of Osgood-Schlatter Disease: A literature review. *The Journal of Orthopaedic Medicine*. 1993; 15:59-63.

11. Brukner P, Khan K. *Clinical Sports Medicine*. New York City, NY: McGraw-Hill Book Company, 1995, pp. 541-560.

12. Gray, J. A survey of injuries to the anterior cruciate ligament of the knee in female basketball players. *International Journal of Sports Medicine*. 1985; 6:314-316.

13. Nilsson, S. Soccer injuries in adolescents. *American Journal of Sports Medicine*. 1978; 6:358-361.

14. Slauterbeck, J. The incidence of anterior cruciate ligament tears in men and women collegiate soccer players. *Orthop. Trans*. 1996; 20:259.

15. Whiteside, P. Men's and women's injuries in comparable sports. *Physician and Sports Medicine*. 1980; 8:130-136.

16. Liu, S. Estrogen affects the cellular metabolism of the anterior cruciate ligament. A potential explanation for female athletic injury. *American Journal of Sports Medicine*. 1997; 25:704-709.

17. Hutchinson, M. Knee injuries in female athletes. *Sports Medicine*. 1995; 19:288-302.

18. Krivickas, L. Lower extremity injuries in college athletes: Relation between ligamentous laxity and lower extremity muscle tightness. *Archives of Physical Medicine and Rehabilitation*. 1996; 77:1139-1143.

19. Johnson, L. Clinical assessment of asymptomatic knees: Comparison of men and women. Arthroscopy: *The Journal of Arthroscopic and Related Surgery*. 1998; 14:347-359.

20. Glick, J. The female knee in athletics. *Physician and Sports Medicine*. 1973; 1:35-37.

21. Powers, J. Characteristic features of injuries in the knees of women. *Clin. Orthop. Rel. Res*. 979; 143:120-124.

22. Lutter, J.M., Lee, V. Exercise in pregnancy. In Pearl AJ, (ed.), *The Female Athlete in Human Kinetics*. Champaign, IL: 1993; p. 81-86.

23. Bennell, K. A prospective study of risk factors for stress injury in female athletes (abstract). In Medicine and science in sports and exercise: *American College of Sports Medicine Annual Meeting Supplement*. 1995; 27:S196.

24. Reeves, K. Treatment of consecutive severe fibromyalgia patients with prolotherapy. *The Journal of Orthopaedic Medicine*. 1994; 16:84-89.

25. Brukner, P. Managing common stress fractures. *The Physician and Sportsmedicine*. 1998; 26:39-47.

26. Bennell, K. The incidence and distribution of stress fractures in competitive track and field athletes: a twelve-month prospective study. *American Journal of Sports Medicine*. 1996; 24:211-217.

27. Bennell, K. A prospective study of risk factors for stress injury in female athletes (abstract). In Medicine and science in sports and exercise: *American College of Sports Medicine Annual Meeting Supplement*. 1995; 27:S196.

28. Myburgh, K. Low bone density is an etiologic factor for stress fractures in athletes. *Annals of Internal Medicine*. 1990; 113:754-759.

29. Drinkwater, B. Bone mineral content of amenorrheic and eumenorrheic athletes. *New England Journal of Medicine*. 1984; 311:277-281.

30. Lloyd, T. Women athletes with menstrual irregularity have increased musculoskeletal injuries. *Med. Sci. Sports Exerc*. 1986; 18:374-379.

31. Bennell, K. Risk factors for stress fractures in female track and field athletes: a retrospective analysis. *Clinical Journal of Sports Medicine*. 1995; 5:229-235.

32. Bennell, K. Risk factors for stress fractures in track and field athletes: a twelve-month prospective study. *American Journal of Sports Medicine*. 1996; 24:810-818.

CHAPTER 8

Be Cautious of X-rays, MRIs, and Surgery

People who come to Caring Medical are quick to show me their x-rays or MRIs. I often ask them "Why did you get this MRI?" The typical response is "because I wanted to see what is wrong with my knee." Wrong answer. You see, an MRI is primarily used by a surgeon to get a patient ready for surgery. An MRI is to *confirm* what the doctor already knows *and* to get the patient ready for surgery. "Were you going to get surgery on your knee?" "No way!" "Then why did you have the MRI?"

The first point of this chapter is to not use x-rays and MRIs to tell you what is wrong with you knee. That is just like agreeing to a "look and see" arthroscopy. Do you really think the orthopedic surgeon is just going to "look and see?" There is nothing wrong with a person going to their general practitioner or orthopedist with knee pain but once something beside physical therapy is ordered, I recommend a second opinion from a doctor who does Prolotherapy. Let's look at the various options open to a traditional doctor to treat your knee pain:

- *Anti-inflammatory medications*
- *Narcotic medications*
- *Cortisone/steroid shot*
- *X-ray/MRI*
- *Arthroscopy/Surgery*

Which one of these available treatments is going to help repair your injured knee? Of course, none of them. As a matter of fact, they do the opposite. All of these treatments will inhibit the healing of your knee and ultimately accelerate the arthritic process. You might ask, "Well, how is getting an x-ray or MRI going to do that?" *Well,* the x-ray will show some jagged cartilage and a bone spur here or there and before you know it you are naked on an operating table and the x-ray findings had nothing to do with your pain and *well* those tissues were shaved during the operation and Voilá! You are left with a meniscus-less knee just ripe for the growth of arthritis. On rare occasions, someone actually does have a completely torn ligament of the knee and needs surgery, but even in these situations I recommend getting a Prolotherapist's second opinion. You would be amazed how many I have seen who on clinical exam have an intact ligament which was called a complete tear by MRI. When the ligament underwent Prolotherapy, the patient/athlete was fine. No surgery needed.

MOST KNEES HAVE SOME SOME DEGENERATION ON X-RAYS.

X-rays will find arthritis. So why get a plain x-ray? Drs. Johnson, Van Dyke, and Green performed a good study of the knee comparing physical examination and x-ray findings on 210 pain-free women and men. The x-rays included the standard knee x-rays of neutral standing PA position, supine, AP, lateral tunnel views and Merchants' views to see underneath the kneecap. Remember these were people who had never experienced any knee complaints. These people considered their knees to be normal. The participants were ages 18 to 85. Here is a summary of the results in these asymptomatic men and women in *Figure 8-1.* [1]

FIGURE 8-1: THE PHYSICAL EXAMINATION AND X-RAY FINDINGS OF ASYMPTOMATIC KNEES

	Women (Percent)	Men (Percent)
PHYSICAL EXAMINATION:		
Normal knee physical examination	4.5	21
Cracking under the kneecap: (Patellofemoral crepitus)	94	45
Cracking on the inside or outside of knee (Medial/lateral compartments)	42	6
Hypermobility to extension	83	48
Asymmetric knees	47	68
X-RAY FINDINGS:		
Evidence of arthritis	84	80
Lateral and medial arthritic findings:		
Scalloping (indentations/erosions)	25	19
Sclerosis (hardening)	40	15
Osteophytes (bony outgrowths)	10	22
ARTHRITIC FINDINGS UNDERNEATH THE KNEE CAP		
(Via the Merchant's view)		
Lateral view position	23	23
Lateral overhang	22	12
Lateral facet sclerosis	49	13
Osteophytes	3	28

Figure 8-1:
This shows how physical examination and x-ray findings can be totally misleading, as people with no symptoms can have significant abnormalities.

The study examined just how "normal" knees that are totally asymptomatic show significant abnormalities on physical examination and on various x-ray studies. The authors noted, "...because patellofemoral crepitus (cracking of the knees) is so common in both symptomatic and asymptomatic volunteers, the importance of this finding must be reevaluated as a surgical indication, as a factor in treatment algorithms, and in practice guidelines, or the inclusion of crepitus as a negative factor in scoring surgical outcomes." Many athletes are told they have chondromalacia patella (cartilage damage underneath the kneecaps) because their knees make noise. They are told that this is causing their pain. They are subjected to frequent scopes and cortisone shots. Athletes, realize cracking of the knees and abnormalities on x-ray is a very common finding. Do not let anyone cortisone you!

The extensive findings on an x-ray showed, "...the use of radiographic evidence alone to establish a diagnosis of patellar subluxation would not be supported by this study." In other words, x-rays cannot tell you that your knee is loose. The study gave yet a few more blows to the orthopedist's desire for arthroscopic and surgical cases by stating, "A presence of general radiographic observations often considered abnormal (scalloping and sclerosis—signs of arthritis) in the lateral patellar radiographic view should lead the physician to use caution when using such findings to determine abnormality or a surgical indication. Minimal increased tibial sub-

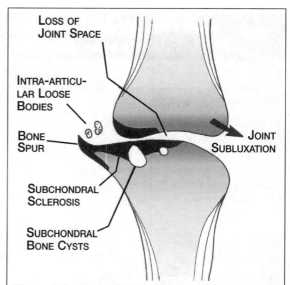

Figure 8-2: General X-Ray Features of Degenerative Joint Disease
Many of the above findings are seen in asymptomatic joints—another reason not to rely on x-rays for diagnosis.

chondral density (sclerosis is a sign of arthritis) is reported to be a radiographic sign of osteoarthritis. Because this was observed in most of these asymptomatic volunteers, this sign alone should not determine the diagnosis of osteoarthritis... In light of this information, surgical indications should be re-evaluated collectively and certainly individually, especially for patellar problems." [1] This study was published in May of 1998. *(See Figure 8-2.)*

MRI OF THE KNEES IN SYMPTOMATIC CHILDREN AND ADULTS

To evaluate the MRIs of adults without any knee symptoms, LaPrade and associates recruited 54 volunteers. This study found that 5.6 percent of asymptomatic volunteers had meniscal tears, but 24 percent had degenerative changes involving the posterior horn of the medial meniscus. [2] The average age of the participant in the study was 28.5 years. The authors stated, "One could assume that the prevalence of asymptomatic findings in an older population would be increased." They are correct in their assumption. Kornick and associates showed that meniscal abnormalities in the asymptomatic population, per MR imaging, increases sharply with age.[3] Sixty-four asymptomatic volunteers were evaluated by MR imaging, looking for meniscal abnormalities. The study showed that in regard to the posterior lateral meniscus during the second decade, 20 percent show abnormalities but by the seventh decade, 60 percent are abnormal. However, for asymptomatic volunteers in their 20s, 62 percent showed abnormalities in the posterior medial meniscus by MRI and, by the age of 70, over 90 percent of the menisci showed these changes. *(See Figure 8-3.)* The significance of these findings is very scary. A 21 year old college football player gets clobbered during a game and has resultant knee pain. The MRI reveals an abnormality in the meniscus and surgery is recommended. How do you know that the MRI finding was not there before the football injury, since 62 percent of young adults have meniscal abnormalities on MRI, yet are without symptoms? Do you see why athletes need a Prolotherapist on their team? Even if a meniscal injury is felt to be the cause of the problem, Prolotherapy is a better option because it is the only one that can potentially proliferate or regenerate the injured tissue.

Part of the reason there are so many "abnormalities" in the menisci in asymptomatic individuals is because structures that attach to the menisci can cause an increased signal in them, which produces the false appearance of a meniscal tear. This was demonstrated in a study in which 109 patients had both arthroscopy and MR imaging of the knee, and the two were correlated.[4] It was found in this study that 42 people (39%) had a normal meniscofemoral ligament attaching onto the lateral meniscus that was appearing on the MR scan as a lateral meniscal tear (high-signal intensity). There are just a lot of studies showing that MRI of the knees is probably going to show an abnormality, regardless if the person has pain or not, so if surgery is contemplated, a second opinion is warranted.

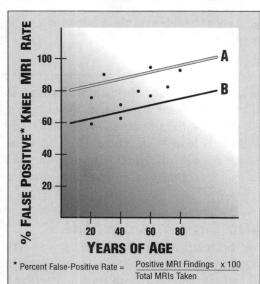

* Percent False-Positive Rate = $\dfrac{\text{Positive MRI Findings} \times 100}{\text{Total MRIs Taken}}$

Figure 8-3: Graph of the Percent False-Positive Knee MRIs of the Medial Meniscus, Findings in Asymptomatic People Relative to Age

The two studies (A & B) show that even by age 20, the number of abnormal MRIs of the knee, in people without any symptoms, is quite substantial. So athletes, beware of arthroscopies that are recommended based solely on MRI data.[3] (A & B studies are discussed in reference number 3.)

Kornick and associates investigated 64 volunteers between the ages of 10 and 74 and found over 25 percent had abnormal signals in their menisci, despite being totally asymptomatic.[3] More distressing is the fact that in another study on children, mean age 12.2 years, that 66 percent showed a high signal intensity within the menisci.[5] A high signal intensity is one of the criterion to diagnose degenerative menisci. This is obviously not abnormal in asymptomatic 12 year olds! The prevalence decreased with age: grade-2 and grade-3 changes were observed in 80 percent of menisci at age 10, in 65 percent at 13 years, and in 35 percent at 15 years. The danger of these findings lies in the fact that there was a tremendously high increased signal rate in the posterior horn of the medial meniscus, in which degeneration and tears are often found. *(See Figure 8-4.)* When a 15 year old football player injures his knee and goes to the orthopedist, what is the doctor going to do? MRI time! What is the MRI going to find?

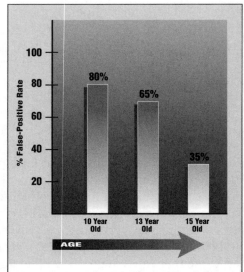

Figure 8-4: False-Positive MRIs of the Knee in Teenagers
Because significant abnormalities show up in the menisci on MRI in teenagers, when no true injury exists, relying on this modality to make a diagnosis is a scary proposition, especially if surgery is contemplated.

Increased signal in the meniscus. What does that mean? Most likely nothing! If the athlete does not get another opinion, he is off for a meniscal shaving, not knowing that shaving the meniscus will increase the pressures on the articular cartilage by up to 700 percent. This will likely lead to significant degenerative arthritis by the time he is in his late 20s and early 30s. No, do not rely on tests for answers. Rely on the thumb. It is more accurate, less expensive, and, of course, quicker.

PROBLEMS WITH CARTILAGE AND CRUCIATES ON MRI

The summary of MRI findings from the main textbook on MRI and sports medicine states, "The MRI imaging of cartilage remains a controversial topic. There is considerable disagreement on the MR appearance of normal cartilage and the accuracy of MR imaging for the detection of the early changes of osteoarthritis."[6] You do not even want to know what studies show on ACL injuries. Well, we are going to tell you anyway. C. Stanitski, M.D., from the Children's Hospital of Michigan, evaluated the correlation among clinical diagnosis, magnetic resonance imaging reports, and arthroscopic findings in 28 patients, aged eight to 15 years (average 14.4 years), with knee injuries. Meniscal, anterior cruciate ligament, and articular surface injuries were evaluated. A highly positive correlation (78.5 percent) was found between clinical examination and arthroscopic findings. A highly negative correlation was found between arthroscopic and magnetic resonance imaging findings and between clinical examinations and magnetic resonance imaging findings. The study showed that accuracy, positive predictive value, negative predictive value, sensitivity, and specificity data were much more favorable from the clinical examination than from magnetic resonance imaging. The author went on to say, "Overall, magnetic resonance imaging diagnoses added little guidance to patient management and at times provided spurious information."[7] This is a nice way of saying that, at least in children and adolescents, many times the MRI scan results are completely and totally false. Listen to these results in this study: Twenty of the 28 patients (71 percent) had either a false-positive or false-negative MRI reading. Six (24 percent) of the 28 patients with arthroscopically documented isolated anterior cruciate ligament tears had false-positive results that indicated the medial meniscus was torn. False-negative MRI reports were seen in 14 of the 28 patients (50 percent); five meniscal lesions, three ACL tears, and six of the fourteen patients with osteochondral loose bodies. The MRIs in these children did not even pick up loose cartilage in the joint, which ranged in size from five to 18 millimeters. The sensitivity of MRI in picking up the ACL, meniscal, and articular cartilage injuries was only 50 percent in this study.[7]

The above results were also confirmed in an active sports medicine practice at the University of Pennsylvania.[8] The study again compared MRI findings to clinical examination in arthroscopically documented pathology. The clinical findings had a 100 percent sensitivity and specificity with the arthroscopic findings, whereas MRI was significantly less accurate. MRI has its most inaccuracies with meniscal lesions.

"Come on, Doctor, surely an MRI is a good test?" Sure it is a good test, if you own stock in an MRI company. Of course we order MRIs. We generally order them if a patient is not responding to Prolotherapy. In all of the patients we have seen for knee problems, probably three to four percent of them required an MRI. Of the three or four percent, perhaps half of these went on to get some kind of surgical procedure. Imagine all of the money that was saved by the rest of the patients getting Prolotherapy, getting rid of their pain, and getting on with life! MRIs are the best noninvasive radiographic tests available, but they cannot, nor can they ever by themselves, determine what is causing the pain. This is the job of the physician. *(See Figure 8-5.)* A physician who does surgery is called a surgeon. A surgeon's bias is to use surgical intervention to treat problems. A conservative doctor's bias is to say that nonsurgical tissues are causing pain. The conservative doctors, such as Prolotherapists, concern themselves primarily with eliminating the pain with nonsurgical methods, regardless if the surgeon said surgery was necessary. If a more conservative option is available, the patient should definitely take it! Prolotherapy is such an option.

You need to hear about two more studies, then we will be done with this chapter. They illustrate three important facts about MRIs, sports, and sports injuries.

MRI VERSUS THE THUMB:
WHICH DO YOU WANT DIAGNOSING YOUR ATHLETIC INJURY?

Figure 8-5

FALE-POSITIVE RATE (CONSERVATIVE ESTIMATE) MRI POSITIVE IN ASYMPTOMATIC MIDDLE-AGED ATHLETE	MRI	THUMB
Lower Back	64	0
Neck	50	0
Shoulder	54	0
Knee	62	0
Cost	$1,200	**Free** (Included in Office Visit)
Time Involved	45 Minutes	45 Seconds
Ability to Reproduce Pain	None	100%
Enjoyment by Clinician	None	Lots
Likelihood of Progression to Surgery	Very High	Very Low

MRIs are great at following the progression of disease. Athletic events, such as running, in and of themselves cause tissue-damage. This is why starting a connective tissue building program is vital to any athlete staying healthy. Even one sports season can cause a significant deterioration in athletes' soft tissues. This is why all athletes need a Prolotherapist on their "P" Team. What happens if an athlete goes out for a jog before getting an MRI of the knee? This is a bad idea—unless you want to ensure that you will get surgery. In one study, asymptomatic volunteers were given MRIs of the knees before and after jogging for 30 minutes. Fifty percent of the knees developed effusions (swelling) after the exercise and 50 percent of them developed increased signal intensity within their menisci! The authors noted, "The results of our study indicate that mild effusions develop acutely within the knee joint after jogging and, further, that associated signal intensity changes appear on MR images of the menisci. The clinical significance of these findings is uncertain. Indeed, the volunteers were without complaints referable to their knees, both before and after jogging, and they were subjected to minimal stress loading only. More pronounced changes may be detected after higher levels of stress such as may occur in marathon runners."[9] We know one thing for sure. This study shows that athletes should do no exercise before getting an MRI! Imagine that! Fifty percent of menisci become degenerated, according to MRI, just by jogging for 30 minutes. This is why MRI findings in structures like the menisci have to be viewed with caution. What about looking at MRIs of the knee before and after a college football season? If 30 minutes of jogging causes such significant changes, what is one football season going to bring? Such a study was done on 17 players in the starting lineup on a major college football team. Only asymptomatic knees were chosen. Increased signal intensity was identified in 10 medial menisci of the 17 subjects during the initial MRI. All of the lateral menisci were normal. At the second examination (one week after the season ended), all 10 of the menisci showed progressive changes. Again, all of the subjects were totally asymptomatic.[10] If the athletes had knee pain, what would have been recommended if NSAIDs failed? Arthroscopy, of course. Remember, arthroscopy is the quickest way for an athlete to get arthritis. What is the quickest way to prevent arthritis? Correct, Prolotherapy. Athletes, Prolo your pain away! This would be a good title for a book...

"Doctor, I cannot get Prolotherapy because my orthopedist said I have a complete ACL tear." How was that determined? "The MRI showed it. I guess I need surgery." Guess again. "MRI studies have not been shown to be accurate in the differentiation of complete and partial ACL tears."[11] This is from "the bible" of MRIs and sports medicine.

The best advice to anyone who has been told they have a complete tendon or ligament tear and that surgery is their only option: run, don't walk, to the office of the best Prolotherapist you can find! When you find a Prolotherapist, check his/her thumb. This will give you confidence that you are at the right place. *(See Figure 8-6.)* Prolotherapists prevent athletes and people with chronic pain from getting surgery. Every day, MRIs are just not that accurate in differentiating a complete from a partial tear. Thus, the only way to tell for sure if a person is a surgical candidate is to fail all the available conservative treatments, including Prolotherapy. If athletes would just hold off on surgery until evaluated and treated with Prolotherapy, there would be a lot less of them needing pain pills, knee replacements, and wheelchairs and canes later in life.

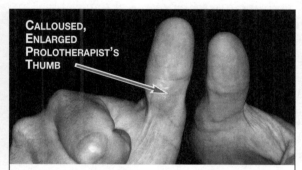

CALLOUSED, ENLARGED PROLOTHERAPIST'S THUMB

Figure 8-6: My Reproducibility Instrument
An experienced Prolotherapist will have a calloused, large thumb from frequent "MRI" testing (positive jump signs) and injections. This is Dr. Hauser's right thumb (on your left).

The most accurate test for the knee, as well as the other joints of the body, is a good history and physical examination. The only MRI that an athlete generally needs is **My Reproducibility Instrument**, the thumb. The thumb is able to move joints and poke on them to reproduce the exact pain. When this is found, the athlete and the doctor do not need any more tests. Prolotherapy is given to the painful areas, which is another test, called the needle test. Generally, after several of these tests have been done, the sports injury is completely healed and the degenerative process stopped. It is for this reason that athletes are saying no to MRIs, because they do not want to have surgery. They are getting second opinions and running to get Prolotherapy. They are learning that there is an alternative to MRIs, arthroscopy, and surgery, and that alternative is the thumb. Poke on the painful area and plunge with the syringe—receive Prolotherapy; it is a better deal than spending the money on an MRI scan which may just lead to unnecessary surgery.

SURGERY IS NO PICNIC.

Obviously in a Prolotherapy practice our patients are no fans of surgery. They typically come to us after surgery did not turn out to be the panacea they thought it would. I often do Prolotherapy after failed knee surgery. This topic is covered in the next chapter. Having seen many devastating effects of surgery please take these points to heart:

1. *Surgery __permanently__ changes anatomy.*
2. *Surgery can leave the knee joint in a very compromised state.*
3. *The rehabilitation time after surgery is extensive.*
4. *Very few elite athletes come back 100% after surgery.*
5. *Surgery is risky.*
6. *Surgery can kill.*

Elite athletes, especially, are under a lot of pressure by the team physician to get surgery. Because of this I think it is important to go over some of the reasons specifically not to get knee surgery.

STUDY SHOWS THERE IS *INCREASED* CONTACT STRESS PRESSURE AFTER MENISCECTOMY.

There have been numerous studies showing that the contact stress pressure on the articular cartilage significantly increases after meniscal removal.[12, 13] One such study showed that after partial meniscectomy, the contact stress pressures increased by 110 percent and after total meniscectomy they increased 200 percent. Their conclusion was expected. "The contact stresses increased in proportion to the amount of meniscus removed.[14] Other studies have shown even greater increases in pressure, causing from a 450 to 600 percent (six times) increase in pressure on the tibia bone and articular cartilage when the meniscus is removed.[15, 16]

Menisci are normally shaved or removed because they are believed to repair so poorly. Menisci, like many of the soft tissues treated with Prolotherapy, have poor blood supply. This is one of the reasons they heal poorly. The best treatment option is to increase the circulation to the damaged menisci. Athletes with meniscal injuries are generally given **RICE** treatment, which dramatically further decreases circulation to the damaged menisci. The **MEAT** protocol and Prolotherapy, on the other hand, improves blood circulation to the damaged area and stimulates repair.

STUDIES SHOW MENISCAL SURGERY ACTUALLY *INCREASES* INJURY.

Repairing a meniscal tear with arthroscopy makes conceptual sense, however, this just does not occur often enough to warrant the procedure. In an animal study, only 38 percent of the meniscal repairs actually healed.[17] To add insult to injury, another study showed that meniscal repair can actually cause a further spreading of the injury to the non-injured meniscal tissue. The authors noted, "It appears that in radial repairs, progressive spreading at the repair site altered normal meniscal geometry and structure, adversely influencing mechanical function."[18] In common language, attempting to repair the area with arthroscopy makes the normal meniscal tissue weaker and further worsens the injury. The authors went on to say, "Meniscal tissue from repaired radial lesions was significantly lower than controls in yield stress, maximum stress, and elastic modulus. The repaired radial meniscal lesions demonstrated abnormal force transmission and energy dissipation behavior qualitatively similar to a complete meniscectomy."[18] This is unbelievable! Repairing a meniscal tear makes the meniscal tissue so weak that it is like having no menisci at all. What a scary thought!

INCOMPLETE HEALING AND FURTHER DETERIORATION RESULT AFTER MENISCAL REPAIR SURGERY

In one large study, where 82 percent of the meniscal injuries were sustained from sporting events, a full 75 percent of the meniscal repairs did not completely heal.[19] The follow-up arthroscopic examinations were done at a mean of 18 months and clinical examinations at 42 months. This is one and a half and three and a half years later, folks. These are not impressive statistics to encourage athletes to undergo meniscal repairs. In this study, in only 18 months, 20 percent of the patients had articular cartilage damage on the tibia and femur that was not present on the initial arthroscopy, but was seen in follow-up arthroscopy. A full 40 percent had deterioration of the articular cartilage under the knee cap.[19] This deterioration occurred over only 18 months! Yet the authors of the paper state that 80 percent of the patients were asymptomatic. But 20 percent of the patients needed further arthroscopic surgery! You see the difference between pain-free and healed? Athletes are being coerced into these procedures that do not repair or heal the injured the tissue. Eighty percent were pain-free while their cartilage was rapidly deteriorating. What is being done to stop this arthritic process? Unless the orthopedist plans to refer the athlete for Prolotherapy, nothing is being done.

MENISCECTOMY CAUSES ARTHRITIS.

Repairing meniscal tears does not work; neither does grafting tissue over the tear. In one study on sheep knees, one group received a total meniscectomy, two groups received different grafts, and the control group received no surgery. Guess which group did better? You guessed it! The virgin knee group that was never probed by a scope fared the best. On follow-up x-ray after only 21 months, the control knees had no arthritis, but the meniscectomized knees had significant arthritis in all the compartments of the knee, as well as the grafted knees. The authors concluded, "Knees undergoing each of the three procedures in our study showed significant degenerative changes when compared with the nonoperated control knees. This would suggest that surgical intrusion into the knee predisposes it to osteoarthritic changes."[20] What a shock!

PARTIAL MENISCECTOMY: MORE ARTHRITIC CHANGES RESULT

Luis Bolano, M.D., and associates at the Oklahoma Center for Athletes and the University of Oklahoma wanted to determine the long-term results of arthroscopic partial meniscectomy. They noted that the short-term results of arthroscopic partial meniscectomy had been excellent-to-good in 80 to 95 percent of patients in the already published studies.[21] What they found surprised them. The patients, many of whom were athletes, were functioning fairly well. Eighty percent experienced satisfactory results, 66 percent maintained their activity levels, but 26 percent decreased their activity levels after the surgery. Despite the apparent success of the surgery, almost all of the patients showed arthritic changes on x-ray. Forty-one percent had advanced arthritis. The authors noted, "The amount of meniscus removed and the type of tear had a significant effect on the radiographic result."[21]

The problem with arthroscopic surgery is that it does not induce the healing of the menisci. The athlete feels better for a while, but the injured tissue remains injured. This causes the arthritic process to start immediately. If left unchecked, the athlete's abilities will decline, symptomatology will increase, and more arthroscopic or orthopedic surgeries will follow. If the athletes want this, then by all means, continue to be scoped. If they want to avoid arthritis, they must see a Prolotherapist and receive Prolotherapy to stimulate the body to heal the menisci and other injured tissue.

THE OUTLOOK IS NOT GOOD FOR POST-SURGICAL ATHLETES.

What is the outlook down the road, 12 to 15 years, for people who have had arthroscopic partial meniscectomies? Not good. In a study of 21 patients who had partial meniscectomy, six needed further meniscal surgery and seven required additional knee surgery. Over 50 percent of the meniscectomized knees needed knee surgery by 12 to 15 years down the road. Eighteen of the 21 patients who underwent meniscectomy had arthritis in the knee. The three with no arthritis were, likely, very inactive people. About 50 percent of the knees, however, had advanced arthritis compared to the non-operated knees. This statement by the authors should be of significance to the athletes, "The activity level of the patients in both groups changed…indicating a downward change from active individual sports, such as tennis, squash, or downhill skiing, to less strenuous physical fitness activities such as cycling, hiking, or cross-country skiing."[22]

Other studies have confirmed similar findings. If no cartilage deterioration occurred before meniscus removal, deterioration will occur after the surgery.[23] Long-term effects of meniscus removal lead to increased contact stresses and subsequent articular cartilage degeneration.[24-27]

144

It is time for athletes to take a stand, even under intense pressure, and say, "The verdict is in: say nope to scope!" Your long-term health may be dramatically altered once the scope enters your knee. At least in meniscal injuries, arthroscopies do not cure anything.

ANTERIOR CRUCIATE LIGAMENT INJURIES

Some of the most horrible words a competitive athlete could hear are, "You have an anterior cruciate ligament tear." All of the treatment options for this condition stink. In the best case scenario, athletes are told that a tendon can replace the ligament and the rehabilitation of this new structure takes a full year. Maybe the athlete will be able to compete again at a later date. In an international sports medicine journal, they put it this way, "The competitive elite athlete who sustains an anterior cruciate ligament (ACL) rupture has few options for treatment. If they wish to continue to compete at the preinjury level, then the only viable option is to undergo an ACL reconstruction. Otherwise, the athlete with an ACL deficient knee is at substantial risk of sustaining subsequent degenerative changes in the knee at a young age.[28]

Ligament injuries in the knee should be treated as potentially serious since they provide for the stability of the knee. They are as common as meniscus injuries and mainly affect athletes involved in contact sports such as football, ice hockey, team handball, basketball, rugby, and also Alpine skiing.[29] Ligament injuries in the knee occur mainly as the result of collisions with opponents during contact sports, but they also occur without body contact, with twisting and other movements that exceed the normal range of motion. The various ligaments of the knee joints cooperate in order to maintain the stability of the joint. The stronger the stresses put on the joint, the greater the degree to which the ligaments are engaged. A ligament combination is often injured because of this fact. Perhaps the most common injury involves the triad of ligaments: the medial meniscus (ligament), medial collateral (ligament), and anterior cruciate (ligament). This occurs because the knee is generally hit from the lateral (outside) side, which forces the knee to buckle inward, injuring those three ligaments. *(See Figure 8-7.)*

ACL TEARS: SOME OF THE WORST INJURIES IMAGINABLE

ACL (anterior cruciate ligament) tears are some of the most common sports injuries. A typical scenario is this: An athlete involved in an

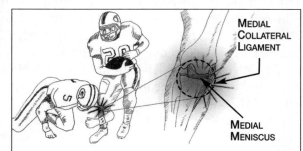

Figure 8-7: Injury to the Medial Meniscus During Contact Sports

A hit on the the knee causing a medial meniscus and medial collateral ligament injury. If the hit is severe enough, the anterior cruciate ligament will also be torn.

145

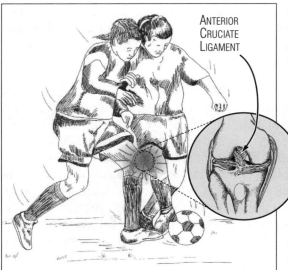

ANTERIOR
CRUCIATE
LIGAMENT

Figure 8-8: Mechanism of Anterior Cruciate Ligament Injury in Agility Sports
When trying to pivot around an opponent, an athlete decelerates and pivots on on a planted foot, causing the ACL injury.

agility sport decelerates and pivots on a planted foot especially when trying to pivot around an opponent, feels a pop in the knee, falls, and is unable to continue play. *(See Figure 8-8.)* Within an hour, the knee swells. X-rays in the emergency room that night are read as negative. The athlete is prescribed **RICE** treatments and an anti-inflammatory medication. After several weeks, the swelling resolves, the pain subsides, and the athlete returns to play. The athlete thinks the doctors and therapists are incredible for the great treatment received. A short time later, the athlete reinjures the knee. The athlete again thinks that he must not be training enough. In reality, the second injury occurred because the original injury never healed. Remember pain relief is not the goal, a healed injury is the goal.

ACL TEARS: TO TREAT OR NOT TO TREAT— THE CHOICES ARE NOT GOOD

ACL tears are so significant because, if left untreated, they have terrible consequences and, if treated, there are bad consequences. It is crucial for the athlete to make the correct choice. Unfortunately the choices are usually between which is the lesser of two evils. If the athlete knows about Prolotherapy, which is the only treatment for ACL tears that actually helps the body repair the injured area, a good choice will be made.

An untreated ACL deficient knee is unstable and arthritis eventually forms. One study following people with ACL tears that were treated nonoperatively showed that 86 percent felt the knee giving way at four-years' follow-up. A full return to unlimited athletic activities was possible for only 14 percent.[30] In another study with about 10 years' follow-up, 78 percent of the knees treated without surgery showed osteoarthritis.[31] Other studies have confirmed that, besides giving way, ACL deficient knees are plagued by swelling and stiffness long term.[32] The most significant finding for most of the studies is that ACL deficient athletes seldom come back to playing their athletics at the same level.

In one study, 72 percent of the athletes had problems with walking, running, turning, cutting, jumping, or climbing stairs 18 months after the injury.[32]

The sad part about ACL injuries is that the injured athlete is usually very young with a full career in the future. Most studies involve athletes who want to return to their athletic events, but few seldom do with this type of injury. In one long-term follow-up study of ACL tears, treated conservatively over a four to 10 year follow-up, only 20 percent of the athletes returned to their preinjury level of athletic activities without restrictions. The rest had arthritis. Eighty-seven percent had evidence of instability on physical examination.[33]

Realize that the conservative treatments the athletes received in the above studies were **RICE**, anti-inflammatories, cortisone shots, physical therapy, and other conservative therapies. They did not receive that treatment that could cure them, which is Prolotherapy. Prolotherapy can cure a partial ACL tear, but not a complete tear. A complete tear requires surgery. Prolotherapy is still helpful in this situation, because the other ligaments around the knee, as well as the joint capsule itself, were at least stretched during the forceful event to the knee that totally disrupted the ACL.

WHAT ABOUT ACL SURGERY?

The standard of care for ACL tears today is surgery. There are various surgical techniques employed in the ACL reconstruction: repair through the patellar defect, arthroscopically-assisted techniques, and the mini-arthrotomy technique. According to one well-known source, "...these techniques all give both excellent and reproducible results."[28] The problem is that the orthopedic surgeons' views on excellent results is different than the athletes' views. The athlete is thinking "I'm going to be back to my sport as good as new as soon as the surgery is over." The orthopedist is thinking, "This athlete doesn't have a chance to be back on that ball field, but the surgery will help stabilize the knee." Poor communication is at the crux of this. The final goals and desired outcomes are never discussed.

ACL reconstruction surgery involves surgically placing a prosthesis or a tendon in the place of the injured ligament. The question to ask is, "Will this surgery allow me to return to athletics?" To answer this question athletes were followed for an average of nine years at the Sports Medicine Facility of Health Sciences at Linkoping University, in Sweden, by Dr. W. Maletius and associates. ACL replacement was performed with Dacron prostheses. In the nine year period, 65 percent of the patients required another arthroscopy. Forty percent had meniscal problems that were treated arthroscopically. At the nine year follow-up only 48 percent of the patients had intact menisci. Forty four percent of the prostheses had ruptured during the follow-up period. Eighty-three percent of the patients had significant arthritic changes on x-ray in the operated knee. The authors concluded, "Based on the functional results of the patients with a ligament in place after nine years, only 14 percent of the original group had acceptable stability and knee function." [34] Some authors have claimed that prosthetic ACL substitution is an "iatrogenic model" of degenerative arthritis in the human knee. [35]

Surgical technique has improved and perhaps the gold standard for ACL reconstruction today is to use the patellar tendon to replace the injured ACL. The surgeon takes some of the patellar tendon and screws it into the femur and tibia bones to simulate an anterior cruciate ligament. The long-term results are better than Dacron prosthesis, but are still not that great. In one five year study of arthroscopic anterior cruciate ligament reconstruction with patellar tendon graft showed that five percent of the patients ruptured their grafts. Of the remaining patients, about 50 percent had symptoms in their knees. Of significance to athletes was that 53 percent of them could perform at the same or a better level at five years post surgery. This means that 47 percent were performing at a lower level of activity. [36] The authors interestingly discussed, "In the literature, there has been a lack of documentation that reconstructing an ACL-deficient knee prevents arthritic changes." [36] In another study following the patients for seven years, a slightly longer period of time, only 46 percent of the athletes could perform at the same level as their preinjury status. In this study 26 percent needed another operative procedure after the ACL reconstruction. [37]

Substituting the real ACL for an artificial one will never be ideal. The tendon grafts have been found to be three to four times stiffer than normal ACLs and artificial graft particles have been shown to cause proliferative arthritis when injected into knees. [38, 39] The athlete's best option is always to first try stimulating the ACL to repair itself. Case reports of complete tears healing without any treatment have been reported in the literature. [40] A much better approach is to receive Prolotherapy for ACL tears. Prolotherapy can be done exactly where the ACL attaches onto the tibia and femur, thereby stimulating the ligament on both ends to proliferate and strengthen. It is only then, by the strengthening of the ACL, will the athlete truly be healed.

SUMMARY REGARDING KNEE ACL SURGERY

For the athlete who puts hope in ACL reconstruction surgery, the road will be a long one. Even if the surgery is successful, a full year of intense rehabilitation is generally needed. Patellar tendon autographs do not achieve full strength evidently until nine months after surgery. [41] An athlete should also realize that a functional knee brace must be worn for 15 to 18 months postoperatively, according to most orthopedists. [42] If the graft is so strong, why would an athlete have to wear a brace? The answer is that the grafts are not that strong. Other researchers have noticed that a high percentage of knees become lax (weak) more than two years postoperatively. [43] The best option for the athlete is to try Prolotherapy to the ACL. Even Prolotherapists are often amazed at how quickly the athlete rockets back once the proliferation of the ligament takes hold.

SURGERY VERSUS PROLOTHERAPY

	SURGERY	PROLOTHERAPY
General anesthesia/ epidural required?	Yes	No
Involves removal of tissue?	Yes	No
Involves placing foreign objects into the body?	Yes	No
Possibility of death	Yes	No
Procedure time?	Hours	Minutes
Rehabilitation time?	Prolonged	None
Cost?	Tens of thousands	Hundreds
Ultimate state of the body?	Weakened	Strengthened
Stimulates body to repair painful area?	No	Yes

Figure 8-9: Prolotherapy versus Surgery

There is no real comparison of Prolotherapy versus surgery, yet athletes are continuously choosing surgery over first trying Prolotherapy for their sports injuries.

PROLOTHERAPY— A MUCH BETTER OPTION

Anyone contemplating surgery should get a second opinion from a Prolotherapist. Often, the surgery can be eliminated by a person getting Prolotherapy. Prolotherapy is a much safer, simpler approach than surgery as shown in *Figure 8-9*.

The animal and human research on Prolotherapy is fascinating. I will just give a few examples of it. For the person desiring to study it in depth, please refer to the books *Prolo Your Pain Away!* and *Prolo Your Sports Injuries Away!*

PROLOTHERAPY STIMULATES LIGAMENT GROWTH.
Y. KING LIU, PH.D.

In 1983, Y. King Liu performed a study using the knee ligament in rabbits.[44] His study was done to confirm Dr. Hackett's earlier work and better quantify the strength of the tissue formed by Prolotherapy. *(See Figure 8-10.)* In this study, a five percent sodium morrhuate solution, an extract of cod liver oil, was injected into the femoral and tibial attachments of the medial collateral ligament, the inside knee ligament.

The ligaments were injected five times and then compared to non-injected ligaments. The results showed that in every case Prolotherapy significantly increased ligamentous mass, thickness, and cross-sectional area as well as the ligament strength. In a six-week period, ligament mass increased by 44 percent, ligament thickness by 27 percent, and the ligament-bone junction strength by 28 percent. This research was yet another attestation to the effectiveness of Prolotherapy, showing that Prolotherapy actually causes new tissue to grow.

I should acknowledge that not all orthopedists are scalpel-happy. Dr. Hildebrand headed up a wonderful research study at the Musculoskeletal Research Center in the Department of Orthopedic Surgery at the University of

THE EFFECTS OF FIVE PROLOTHERAPY TREATMENTS TO THE MEDIAL COLLATERAL LIGAMENT

	Prolotherapy-Injected Ligaments	Saline-Injected Ligaments (Control)	% Change
Ligament Mass (mg)	132.2	89.7	44
Ligament Thickness (mm)	1.01	0.79	27
Ligament Mass Length (mg/mm)	6.45	4.39	47
Junction Strength (N)	119.1	93.5	28

Figure 8-10: The Effects of Six Prolotherapy Treatments to the Medial Collateral Ligament
Prolotherapy causes a statistically significant increase in ligament mass and strength as well as bone-ligament junction strength.

Pittsburgh, which won the 1997 O'Donoghue Sports Injury Research Award. They did not know it, but they were researching Prolotherapy of the knee in rabbits. They injected completely torn rabbit medial collateral ligaments (MCL) with various proliferants, including platelet-derived growth factor (PDGF). The MCLs were completely torn by surgery. What they did not know was that they were proving that Prolotherapy could help complete ligament tears repair themselves. They then compared the uninjured MCL with the injured MCL treated by Prolotherapy. They performed only one session of Prolotherapy and then sacrificed the animals at six weeks (the correct time period to allow the Prolotherapy to work). They did the study because of the high incidence of knee ligament injuries and the controversy concerning the treatment. They noted that even with the use of different treatment methods, such as suture repair or early motion, normal ligament properties were not restored in the MCL.[45]

It is significant that the researchers noted that within one or two days after the surgery and subsequent Prolotherapy all rabbits resumed normal cage activity. They had surgery to injure the ligaments by complete transection (type 3 ligament injury). Prolotherapy to the injury site allowed the rabbits to quickly resume normal activity. Only one Prolotherapy treatment was given to the rabbits in these complete ligament tears. The Prolotherapy group showed statistically-significant increases in ligament mass and cross-sectional area. Some of the cross-sectional areas in the Prolotherapy group increased by over 200 percent. The strength of the ligament tissue also increased by 50 percent in only six weeks. The study also confirmed that the stronger the proliferant, the more growth of tissue occurred. *(See Figure 8-11.)*

Feelings of weakness, pain, or cracking in the knees should be treated with Prolotherapy. Because the knee is a weight-bearing joint and is unique in that

PROPERTY	CONTROL	PDGF Low Dose	PDGF High Dose	% INCREASE by High Dose Proliferant
Ultimate load (N) (Ligament strength)	83.7	119.4	130.2	55
Energy Absorbed (J) (Energy required to cause ligament failure)	125	350	380	300
Ultimate Elongation (mm) (Amount of ligament lengthening prior to failure)	4.0	4.7	5.6	40

Figure 8-11: Effect of Prolotherapy on Complete MCL Tears
The proliferant, platelet-derived growth factor (PDGF), injected into the MCL after transection causes a significant increase in ligament strength in all aspects measured.

it involves four bones (tibia, femur, fibula, and patella) instead of the usual two, like the hip, it is very vulnerable to injury. The fact that it is out in the open to be clipped also puts it at increased risk for injury. A joint such as the hip is snugly hidden in its socket. An injury to any structure around the knee has a cascade effect to cause the other structures of the knee to start to deteriorate. This is why knee arthritis is so common in anyone who has had previous knee surgery or injury.

PROLOTHERAPY IMPROVES DEGENERATED KNEES.

Kenneth D. Reeves, M.D., headed up a study on using Prolotherapy for knee osteoarthritis with or without ACL laxity.[46] In this study the patients with knee arthritis received three bimonthly sessions of Prolotherapy. The study found statistical improvement in pain, swelling, buckling episodes and knee flexion range. By one year, the Prolotherapy-treated knees improved in pain (44% decrease), swelling complaints (63% decrease), knee buckling frequency (85% decrease), and in flexion range (14% increase). Analysis of blinded radiographic readings of 0- and 12-month films revealed stability of all radiographic variables except for two variables which improved with statistical significance. (lateral patellofemoral cartilage thickness and distal femur width) This study confirmed that ACL ligament and cartilage repair was possible in humans with Prolotherapy.

SUMMARY

X-rays and MRIs are done frequently to "diagnose" a knee problem. The danger of this approach is that the degeneration found on these scans can lead to arthroscopy and other orthopedic surgeries. These procedures often leave the patient's knee in a weakened state.

A better approach when x-rays, MRIs, surgeries, or for that matter NSAIDs or cortisone shots are considered is for the person to run (don't walk out of the doctors office) to get a second opinion from a Prolotherapist. Prolotherapy stimulates the body to repair the injured knee and can often prevent a person from needing a knee surgery. Prolotherapy has been shown to stimulate ligament repair and reverse the arthritic process. It is for this reason that many people and athletes with knee pain are realizing that the best approach is to Prolo their knee pain away! ■

BIBLIOGRAPHY

1. Johnson, L. Clinical assessment of asymptomatic knees: Comparison of men and women. Arthroscopy: *The Journal of Arthroscopic and Related Surgery.* 1998; 14:347-359.

2. Erkintalo, M. Development of degenerative changes in the lumbar intervertebral disk: results of a prospective MR imaging study in adolescents with and without low back pain. *Radiology.* 1995; 196:529-533. (38)

3. Kornick, J. Meniscal abnormalities in the asymptomatic population at MR imaging. *Radiology.* 1990; 177:463-465.

4. Vahey, T. MR imaging of the knee: pseudotear of the lateral meniscus caused by the meniscofemoral ligament. *American Journal of Radiology.* 1990; 154:1237-1239.

5. Takeda, Y. MRI high-signal intensity in the menisci of asymptomatic children. *The Journal of Bone and Joint Surgery.* 1998; 80B:463-467.

6. Stoller, D. *Magnetic Resonance Imaging in Orthopaedics and Sports Medicine.* Second Edition. Philadelphia, PA: Lippincott-Raven. 1997, 91.

7. Stanitski, C. Correlation of arthroscopic and clinical examinations with magnetic resonance imaging findings of injured knees in children and adolescents. *American Journal of Sports Medicine.* 1998; 26:2-6.

8. Gelb, H. Magnetic resonance imaging of knee disorders: Clinical value and cost-effectiveness in a sports medicine practice. *American Journal of Sports Medicine.* 1996; 24:99-102.

9. Kursunoglu-Brahme, S. Jogging causes acute changes in the knee joint: an MR study in normal volunteers. *American Journal of Radiology.* 1990; 154:1233-1235.

10. Reinig, J. Progression of meniscal degenerative changes in college football players: evaluation with MR imaging. *Radiology.* 1991; 181:255-257.

11. Stoller, D. *Magnetic Resonance Imaging in Orthopaedics and Sports Medicine.* Second Edition. Philadelphia, PA: Lippincott-Raven. 1997, 330.

12. Ahmed, A. In vitro measurement of static pressure distribution in synovial joints. Part 1: Tibial surface of the knees. *Journal of Biomechanical Engineering.* 1983; 105:216-225.

13. Brown, T. In vitro contact stress distributions on the femoral condyles. *Journal of Orthopedic Research.* 1984; 2:190-199.

14. Baratz, M. Meniscal tears: The effect of meniscectomy and of repair on intra-articular contact areas and stress in the human knee. *American Journal of Sports Medicine.* 1986; 14:270-274.

15. Radin, E. Role of the menisci in the distribution of stress in the knee. *Clinical Orthopedics.* 1984; 185:290-294.

16. Seedom, B. Transmission of the load in the knee joint with special reference to the role of the menisci: *Part 1. Eng Med.* 1979; 8:220-228.

17. Cabaud, H. Medial meniscus repairs. *American Journal of Sports Medicine.* 1981; 9:129-134.

18. Newman, A. Mechanics of the healed meniscus in a canine model. *American Journal of Sports Medicine.* 1989; 17:164-175.

19. Rubman, M. Arthroscopic repair of meniscal tears that extend into the avascular zone. *American Journal of Sports Medicine.* 1998; 26:87-95.

20. Edwards, D. Radiographic changes in the knee after meniscal transplantation. *American Journal of Sports Medicine.* 1996; 24:222-229.

21. Bolano, L. Isolated arthroscopic partial meniscectomy. *American Journal of Sports Medicine.* 1993; 21:432-437.

22. Maletius, W. The effect of partial meniscectomy on the long-term prognosis of knees with localized, severe chondral damage. *American Journal of Sports Medicine.* 1996; 24:258-262.

23. Cox, J. The degenerative effects of partial and total resection of the medial meniscus in dogs' knees. *Clinical Orthopedics.* 1975; 109:178-183.

24. Allen, P. Later degenerative changes after medial meniscectomy. *Journal of Bone and Joint Surgery.* 1984; 66B:666-671.

25. Appel, H. Late results after meniscectomy in the knee joint. *Acta Orthop Scand* (Suppl). 1970, pg. 133.

26. Tapper, E. Late results after meniscectomy. *Journal of Bone and Joint Surgery.* 1969; 51A:517-526.

27. Veth, R. Clinical significance of knee joint changes after meniscectomy. *Clinical Orthopedics.* 1985; 198:56-60.

28. Shelbourne, K. Anterior cruciate ligament injury. *Sports Medicine.* 1994; 17:132-140.

29. Peterson, L. *Sports Injuries.* Chicago, IL. Year Book Medical Publishers. 1983; pp. 296-299.

30. Hawkins, R. Follow-up of the acute nonoperated isolated anterior cruciate ligament tear. *American Journal of Sports Medicine.* 1986; 4:205-210.

31. McDaniel, W. Untreated ruptures of the anterior cruciate ligament: A follow-up study. *Journal of Bone and Joint Surgery.* 1980; 62A:696-705.

32. Buckley, S. The natural history of conservatively treated partial anterior cruciate ligament tears. *American Journal of Sports Medicine.* 1989; 17:221-225.

33. Pattee, G. Four to ten year follow-up of unreconstructed anterior cruciate ligament tears. *American Journal of Sports Medicine.* 1989; 7:430-435.

34. Maletius, W. Long-term results of anterior cruciate ligament reconstruction with a Dacron prosthesis. *American Journal of Sports Medicine.* 1997; 25:288-293.

35. Klein, W. Synovitis and artificial ligaments. *Arthroscopy.* 1992; 8:116-124.

36. Otto, D. Five year results of single-incision arthroscopic anterior cruciate ligament reconstruction with patellar tendon autograft. *American Journal of Sports Medicine.* 1998; 26:181-188.

37. Bach, B. Arthroscopically assisted anterior cruciate ligament reconstruction using patellar tendon autograft. *The American Journal of Sports Medicine.* 1998; 26:20-29.

153

38. Noyes, F. Biochemical analysis of human ligament grafts used in knee-ligament repairs and reconstructions. *The Journal of Bone and Joint Surgery.* 1984; 66:344-352.

39. Olson, E. The biochemical and histological effects of artificial ligament wear particles: In vitro and in vivo studies. *The American Journal of Sports Medicine.* 1988; 16:558-602.

40. Kurosaka, M. Spontaneous healing of a tear of the anterior cruciate ligament. *The Journal of Bone and Joint Surgery.* 1998; 80A:1200-1203.

41. Clancy, W. Anterior and posterior cruciate ligament reconstruction in rhesus monkeys. *Journal of Bone and Joint Surgery.* 1981; 63A:1270-1284.

42. Wasilewski, S. Effect of surgical timing on return to sports activity after significant knee injuries. *Sports Medicine.* 1994; 18:156-161.

43. Barber-Westin, S. The effect of rehabilitation and return to activity on anterior-posterior knee displacements after anterior cruciate ligament reconstruction. *American Journal of Sports Medicine.* 1993; 21:264-270.

44. Liu, Y. An in situ study of the influence of a sclerosing solution in rabbit medial collateral ligaments and its junction strength. *Connective Tissue Research.* 1983; 2:95-102.

45. Hildebrand, K. The effects of platelet-derived growth factor-BB on healing of the rabbit medial collateral ligament. *American Journal of Sports Medicine.* 1998; 26:549-554.

46. Reeves, K. Hassanein, K. Randomized prospective double-bllind placebo-controlled study of dextrose prolotherapy for knee osteoarthritis with or without ACL laxity. In the journal *Alternative Therapies.* March 2000; vol. 6, no. 2 pp. 68-80.

CHAPTER 9

Prolotherapy after Failed Knee Surgery

"If you go to a retired (football) players' convention, there are older retirees who walk around like Maryland crabs," says Miki Yaras-Davis, director of benefits for the NFL Players Association. "It's an orthopedic surgeon's dream. I'm surprised the doctors aren't standing outside the door handing out their cards.[1]
—Sports Illustrated, May 7, 2001

WHEN THE STAKES ARE HIGH, SO ARE THE EXPECTATIONS.

In professional football, the average length of a player's career is a remarkably short four years. Compared to the other major sports, it is by far, the least amount of career years.

The chance to be injured playing, practicing or even training for a National Football League (NFL) game is obviously high. Anyone who has not witnessed an NFL game in person cannot truly understand the beatings some players take or how some players maximize their body's adrenaline "fight or flight syndrome," capabilities to an extreme. For instance, in running back a kick off for a touchdown, a player will sprint some 100 yards in 10 seconds (a fantastic feat in itself) while cutting, darting and decking 250-300 pound men determined to punish him with a massive tackle.

So the risks of injury are high, the money invested by an owner into a player is high, the expectation of performance from the player is high, and so is the expectation of medical care the player expects to receive when injured-but who's expectation is this? The players or the teams?

The physician who manages and determines what course of treatment an injured professional athlete receives is obviously the team physician. The team physician of course is an employee or "contractor" to the team and paid by the team. Because the team physician is paid by the team, this possibly leads to some players suspecting that it may be the team's best interests will prevail, not their own.

Doctors should tell you that you shouldn't play or practice. He should take responsibility. But he's the team doctor, and his No. 1 loyalty is to the team.[2]
—Ex-NFL player Don Davey

So with a poor track record of putting a large number of players back onto the field in a condition somewhat close to that prior to the injury, players will get mad at their doctors. Some will even file lawsuits against their teams and their team's doctors because of this.

(The determination of whether a player can successfully sue a team physician was at question in a recent lawsuit by an NFL player. It was ruled that the player could not sue the team physicians for complications after knee surgery because the physicians were his co-employees. In this case, the player would only be entitled to worker's compensation. It should be noted that the player's unions of the major sports fought to have the doctors in this case termed independent contractors so the player could sue.)

There are cases where—not only in football, but in other sports—a player sued a team and the team physician for what they thought were questionable surgeries. Some players, while not resorting to legal action, aired the voices to the media.

> "We're just skeptical of doctors, period." Dolphins guard Jamie Nails said, "You try to trust them. Try. But we tend to know our bodies better than they do." [3]

But again, to be fair, it is easy for a player to become frustrated and angry when medicine does not work for them as judged by the aforementioned very short career expectation. It can be well argued that orthopedic sports medicine does not do well for an injured football player. But then, in the high stakes world of professional sports, where a player's career is at stake and where an owner can be out millions of dollars for a player who can no longer perform, a lot rides on a medical outcome being successful. Unfortunately, we know there are plenty of times the player has to retire or play at a level far below that to which he and his fans are accustomed.

Recently a football player sued his team and team doctor. The contention by the player was that the team doctor may have performed an "extended" surgery, a procedure more than that agreed to the player. The player said that his career was over because of this surgery and that some of his teammates will back up his claim with their own that the doctor performed other "extra" procedures during surgeries.

Whether the player is correct or not does not matter in this case. What does matter is that the player believed that the surgery ended his career. Now what about other players around the league? In the back of their mind, might they not think that surgery has its risks? One can at least be sure of the fact that for some players it *was* the surgery that ended their careers.

WHY, THEN, DON'T MORE ELITE ATHLETES GET PROLOTHERAPY?

Because there is an underlying belief that the quickest way back to the game is through surgery—and team physicians are of course surgeons.

For some reason athletes are still trusting of their teams and team physicians. Since the team physicians are orthopedic surgeons they are not going to recommend Prolotherapy. Orthopedic Surgeons are surgeons, they love to do surgery. They have no expertise in Prolotherapy except to tell athletes it isn't for them. The athlete unfortunately doesn't realize the orthopedist has very little knowledge about Prolotherapy, so they shouldn't be giving an opinion about it.

The athlete who wants to know if they are a good Prolotherapy candidate needs to see a Prolotherapist. Only a physician experienced in Prolotherapy would be able to tell an athlete whether their injuries can be treated successfully with Prolotherapy. Prolotherapy can be used for almost all athletic injuries. The most common injuries treated with Prolotherapy are tendon, ligament, menisci, and cartilage weakness. For the athlete who has a structure that won't completely repair with exercise and rehabilitation, Prolotherapy is almost always the way to go. Prolotherapy to the affected area can stimulate the repair. For the elite athlete this means back to training quickly. It means that they will soon be back into the game.

WHEN IN DOUBT, THINK PROLOTHERAPY.

As explained many times in this book, when in doubt, think Prolotherapy. If you are not sure of a doctor's opinion, get a second opinion from a Prolotherapist. Even if the doctor says knee surgery is absolutely necessary. Well is it an emergency? Can it wait a day? If so, then contact a Prolotherapist. When in doubt, think Prolotherapy. *(See Figure 9-1.)*

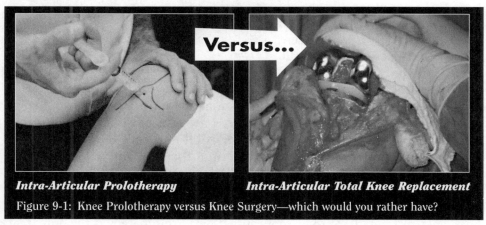

Intra-Articular Prolotherapy   *Intra-Articular Total Knee Replacement*

Figure 9-1: Knee Prolotherapy versus Knee Surgery—which would you rather have?

KNEE PROLOTHERAPY VERSUS KNEE SURGERY— WHICH WOULD YOU RATHER HAVE?

The complications of orthopedic surgery are significant and frequent. Most are outlined in the section on arthroscopy. The ligament grafts are profoundly weakened about eight weeks after surgery. At this time their strength is about 10 percent of its initial strength! It is only 50 percent of initial strength after one year. In two to three years the grafts are at their strongest, and then, less than their initial strength.[4] Compare this to one study where ligament strength was measured after a six-week period of doing Prolotherapy on knee ligaments. The results showed that in every case Prolotherapy increased ligamentous mass, thickness, and cross-sectional area as well as the ligament strength. Prolotherapy in a six-week period increased ligament mass by 44 percent, ligament thickness by 27 percent, and the ligament-bone junction strength by 28 percent.[5] There are other techniques for ACL problems, including artificial grafts. These artificial grafts (e.g., Gortex) lead to particularly poor results with very high complications![6,7] Arthrofibrosis (a scarred, painful, stiff, knee with limited use) followed arthroscopic ACL reconstruction in 10 percent of the cases, when associated with the repair of a torn meniscus![8]

In an Australian study, patients were followed up after 7.4 years. Fifty-seven percent had pain on exertion. There was an overall significant deterioration of the anterior-posterior stability of the knee, indicating a failure of the ligament graft integrity with time.[9] In another study of patients followed for two to seven years after surgery, seven percent of the grafts failed and another 26 percent had only "fair" results.[10]

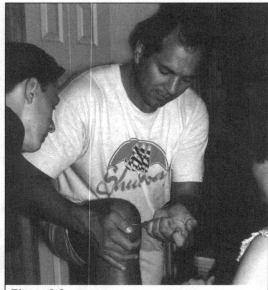

Figure 9-2:
Dr. Rodney Van Pelt takes the phrase, "Physician, Heal Thyself" very seriously...

When Prolotherapy is given, the joint stability is restored and painless function returns! Because of the ligaments' location outside the capsule, these injections must be directed specifically at the ligament attachments to bone at all four ends of the cruciates, if they are both injured. A simple injection into the joint will not do the same thing, although this may be needed as well if arthritis is present from the injury. Prolotherapy is a simple solution for a myriad of seemingly complex knee problems. They all involve injury to the soft tissues of the knee (meniscus, cartilage, ligaments, or tendons) at their root cause. Since Prolotherapy is the only treatment that specifically re-grows soft tissues at the exact site of injury, it is effective for the vast majority of knee conditions in athletes. *(See Figure 9-2.)*

PROLOTHERAPY AND THE SURGICALLY FAILED KNEE

On an initial consultation I will tell patients that Prolotherapy stimulates the body to repair painful areas. If this is true that it is obviously going to help a lot of different conditions. It doesn't matter if the damage to the knee came from a sports injury, NSAID, cortisone shot, or surgical procedure. The tissue always heals the same way. If a joint and/or its structures are damaged, weakened, torn, or degenerated the treatment they need is Prolotherapy. In many respects— does the person has a choice? Choose either further degeneration or regeneration with Prolotherapy. *(See Figure 9-3.)*

When a person has surgery on the knee, typically they are left with less meniscal tissue and greater stresses on the articular cartilage. In these cases physicians who do Prolotherapy will inject Prolotherapy solution into the joint to stimulate repair. Sometimes stronger proliferants will used such as Growth

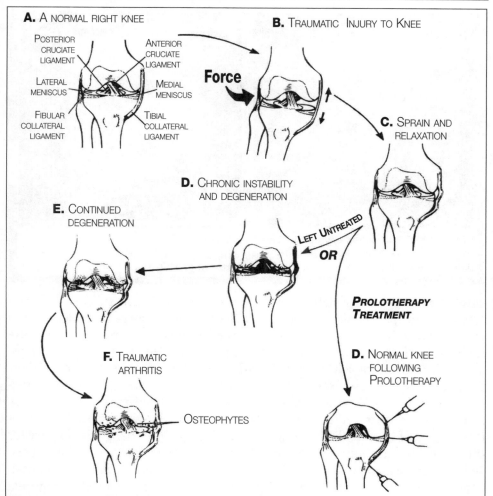

Figure 9-3: How Soft Tissue Injury Leads to Degenerative Arthritis
Ligaments become sprained following trauma. When healing does not occur, the ligaments become relaxed, resulting in chronic instability and degeneration from meniscal and articular cartilage degeneration. When left untreated, post-traumatic "arthritis" or degenerative osteoarthritis follows. This degenerative process can be prevented with appropriate intervention through Prolotherapy.

Hormone. The cartilage cells have Growth Hormone receptors on them. In terms of repair, cartilage is generally slower to heal then the other tissues typically treated with Prolotherapy; therefore it may take more time and treatment sessions. With enough treatments the articular cartilage can and does repair. **(See Figure 9-4.)**

SUMMARY

Prolotherapy is useful for a wide range of sports knee injuries and is a much better option than cortisone shots, arthroscopy, and especially surgery. In many

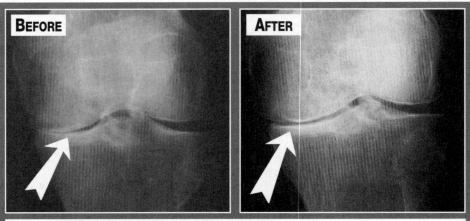

Figure 9-4: Prolotherapy Stimulates Cartilage Repair
Prolotherapy can stimulate not only the repair of ligament, tendon, muscle, and menisci tissue but also cartilage, as evidenced by the increase in joint space narrowing.

cases it can save the athlete from the risks associated with surgery, the long rehabilitation period after surgery, and the failures of surgery. Athletes often end up with arthritic knees, not because they exercised too much, but because their original knee injuries were not completely healed. This is often because athletes are given the **RICE** protocol with anti-inflammatories to decrease their pain. If this does not work, cortisone shots, arthroscopy, and other surgical recommendations are soon to follow. These are definitely decreasing the healing. Athletes are encouraged to use the **MEAT** protocol along with specific physiotherapy, and if needed, Prolotherapy after an injury. Prolotherapy is effective for the myriad of knee injuries, because all of them involve injuries to the soft tissue structures (meniscus, articular cartilage, tendons, and ligaments). Prolotherapy is also successful for the person who experienced suboptimal results with knee surgery. Because the degenerative process is the same, no matter what the cause, Prolotherapy can stimulate the areas to repair that were injured with surgery. Athletes and those previously surgerized are finally realizing that they can get back to sports because of the healing powers of Prolotherapy. Prolotherapy is effective for the myriad of knee injuries because all of them involve injuries to the soft tissue structures including the menisci, articular cartilage, tendons, and ligaments. With Prolotherapy the athlete and those desiring to be active can heal sports injuries and other knee pains permanently, naturally, and safely! ▪

BIBLIOGRAPHY

1. *The Wrecking Yard* by William Nack, special reporting by Lester Munson
   http://sportsillustrated.cnn.com/si_online/news/2002/09/11/wrecking_yard/
   Accessed February 1, 2004

2. *NFL medical policies under scrutiny,* Pete Prisco, SportsLine.com, Nov. 13,
   2002, http://cbs.sportsline.com/nfl/story/5886079

3. *Doctoring the truth in the NFL, Miami Herald,* Oct. 25, 2002 by Dan Le Batard
   http://www.miami.com/mld/miami/sports/4363752.htm

4. Tria, A. *Ligaments of the Knee.* New York, NY: Churchill Livingstone Inc.
   1995, p. 167.

5. Liu, Y. An in situ study of the influence of a sclerosing solution in rabbit medial
   collateral ligaments and its junction strength. *Connective Tissue Research.*
   1983; 2:95-102.

6. Paulos, L. The Gore-tex anterior cruciate ligament prosthesis. A long-term
   follow-up. *American Journal of Sports Medicine.* 1992; 20:246-252.

7. Letsch, R. Replacement of the anterior cruciate ligament by a PET prosthesis
   (Trevira extra-strength as a salvage procedure in chronically unstable
   previously operated knee joints). *Unfallchirurgie.* 1994; 20:293-301.

8. Austin, K. Complications of arthroscopic meniscal repair. *American Journal
   of Sports Medicine.* 1993; 21:864-868.

9. Cross, M. Acute repair of injury to the anterior cruciate ligament. A long-term
   follow-up. *American Journal of Sports Medicine.* 1993; 21:128-131.

10. Noyes, F. Reconstruction of the anterior ligament with human allograft.
    Comparison of early and later results. *Journal of Bone and Joint Surgery*
    (American) 1996; 78: 524-537.

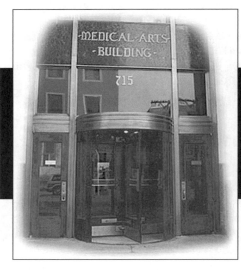

CARING MEDICAL AND REHABILITATION SERVICES

NATURAL MEDICINE CENTER

Therapies offered at Caring Medical

- Biological Aging Measurement
- Bio-oxidative Therapies (Oxygen Therapies)
- Chelation Therapy
- Cryotherapy
- Enzyme Replacement Therapy
- Herbal Help
- Huneke Neural Therapy

- Hyperthermia
- Infrared Coagulation
- Insulin Potentiation Therapy (IPT)
- Mesotherapy
- Metabolic Typing
- Natural Gynecology
- Natural Hormone Replacement Therapy for Men and Women
- NeuroCranial Restructuring

- Nutritional/Herbal Regimes
- Ozone Therapy
- Photoluminescense
- Prolotherapy
- Radiofrequency
- Therapeutic Skin Care Analysis and Treatment

**Care for the *Whole* Person.
Your Health Concerns Addressed in a Comprehensive
Natural Medicine Environment.**

*Would you like to contact us or make an appointment?
To find out more, call now!*

Call now: 708-848-7789 or e-mail us at: info@caringmedical.com for more information.

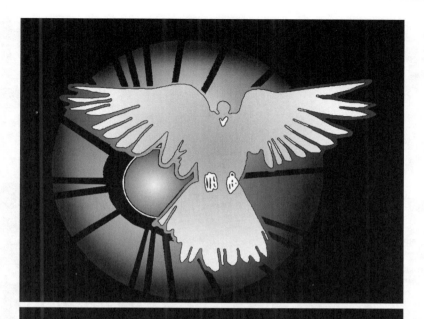

FOR MORE INFORMATION

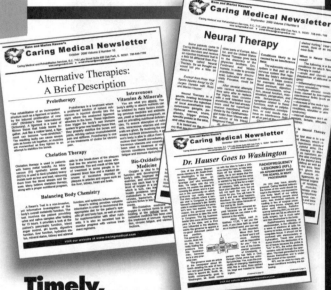

George S. Hackett AMA Presentations

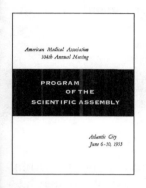

AMERICAN MEDICAL ASSOCIATION
104TH ANNUAL MEETING
PROGRAM OF THE SCIENTIFIC ASSEMBLY
ATLANTIC CITY, JUNE 6-10, 1955

DIAGNOSIS AND TREATMENT OF BACK DISABILITIES
GEORGE S. HACKETT, CANTON, OHIO

"Relaxation of the posterior ligaments of the spine and pelvis is the most frequent cause of back pain and disability. Diagnosis is made by trigger point pressure and confirmed by injecting an anaesthetic within the ligament. The local and referred pain are immediately reproduced and disappear within two minutes. The patient's confidence is established. Treatment consists of injection of a proliferant within the ligament which stimulates the production of bone and fibrous tissue, which becomes permanent. New areas of referred pain in the groin, buttock, and extremities have been identified during the past 16 years while making over 3,000 injections within the ligaments of 563 patients, with 82 percent considering themselves cured. Ages range from 15 to 81 years. Longest duration before treatment was 49 years; the average was 4 and a half years. X-rays of animal experiments carried out over two years reveal the proliferation of abundant permanent tissue at the fibro-osseous junction."

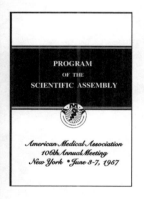

AMERICAN MEDICAL ASSOCIATION
106TH ANNUAL MEETING
PROGRAM OF THE SCIENTIFIC ASSEMBLY
NEW YORK, JUNE 3-7, 1957

PAIN, REFERRED PAIN AND SCIATICA IN BACK DIAGNOSIS AND TREATMENT
GEORGE S. HACKETT, MERCY HOSPITAL, CANTON, OHIO

"Referred pain into the extremities and sciatica results more often from relaxed ligaments of unstable joints than from all other causes combined. Referred pain areas into the groin, lower abdomen, genitalia, buttock and extremities to as far as the toes from articular ligaments that support the lumbar and pelvic joints have been established from observations while making over 10,000 intraligamentous injections in the diagnosis and treatment of 1,207 patients during the past 18 years. Articular ligament relaxation has been found to be the cause of more chronic low back disability than from any other entity. The trigger points of pain of specific disabled ligaments have been established. In diagnosis, knowledge of the referred pain areas directs attention to specific ligaments, and in conjunction with the trigger points of pain, enables the physician to accurately locate the cause of the disability. Ninety percent of the patients with joint instability are cured by the intraligamentous injection of a proliferating solution which stimulates the production of new bone and fibrous tissue cells to permanently strengthen the ligaments."

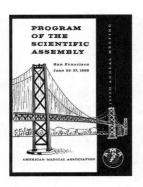

AMERICAN MEDICAL ASSOCIATION
107TH ANNUAL MEETING
PROGRAM OF THE SCIENTIFIC ASSEMBLY
SAN FRANCISCO, JUNE 23-27, 1958

CERVICAL WHIPLASH INJURY
GEORGE S. HACKETT, CANTON, OHIO

"Chronic whiplash cervical pain has its origin within incompetent occipital tendons and cervical articular ligaments which stretch under normal tension and permit an over-stimulation of the nonstretchable sensory nerve fibrils at the fibro-osseous junction. It results in headache and specific referred pain areas to as far as the eyes, temples, and fingers. The diagnosis is invariably confirmed by intraligamentous needling with an anesthetic solution. Eighty-two percent of 1,656 patients throughout 19 years considered themselves permanently cured by Prolotherapy (rehabilitation of an incompetent structure by the proliferation of new cells—bone and fibrous tissue 'weld')."

The information in this appendix is from abstracts of Dr. Hackett's presentations and is used with permission of the American Medical Association, Chicago, Illinois. ▪

Prolotherapy Referral List

While Prolotherapy is a technique that is still relatively unknown, it is gaining popularity. Many folks from around the country desire to come to Caring Medical for their Prolotherapy because of our years of experience. If you or a loved one needs Prolotherapy, I or one of my associates would love to treat you.

Ross A. Hauser, M.D.
Caring Medical & Rehabilitation
Services, S.C.
715 Lake Street, Suite 600
Oak Park, Illinois, 60301
708-848-7789
www.caringmedical.com
drhauser@caringmedical.com

INTERNET PROLOTHERAPY REFERRAL LIST

We believe that the best site on the internet for Prolotherapy referrals is **www.getprolo.com**. On this site, you will find doctors all over the country who do Prolotherapy.

GET PROLOTHERAPY INFORMATION DIRECTLY SENT TO YOUR COMPUTER!

Would you like to know what Caring Medical is doing these days? Subscribe to the Caring Medical Newsletter and find out! To subscribe to our weekly e-newsletters, go to this link: caringmedical.com/media/subscriptions.asp.

FOR FURTHER INFORMATION, PLEASE SEE:

www.caringmedical.com
www.prolonews.com
www.sportsprolo.com

IF YOU DESIRE THE LATEST PROLOTHERAPY INFORMATION:

The site GetProlo.com (www.getprolo.com) is the most comprehensive site for Prolotherapy resources in the world. You can check availability in your area, or research another location. Find out when new doctors are added, read general articles, case histories, medical peer-reviewed articles and catch up on Prolotherapy news.

TEACHING TAPES FOR PHYSICIANS

Teaching tapes that illustrate the technique of Prolotherapy, by David Brewer, M.D., Ross Hauser, M.D., Gustav A. Hemwall, M.D., and Jean-Paul Ouellette, M.D., can be ordered by calling 1-800-RX-PROLO. ■

Actual Patient Letters

"I had my knee go out on me over a period of three or four months. It was so bad I spent two weeks in our recliner with my leg propped up and straight. I could not bend my knee and the pain was unbearable. I finally considered going to a doctor about my knee. I went to an orthopedic surgeon who said, after looking at the x-rays, that I had torn cartilage and needed surgery. I scheduled the surgery and started asking other people about similar problems. When I called a customer to inform them I couldn't do their remodeling job they told me about Prolo. I cancelled my surgery and got an appointment in July to have my knee done at Caring Medical. The pain is gone and I can do almost anything I want. I just had my second treatment and expect to be fine."

*– Sam Smithson**

"Amazing! That's what your Prolotherapy has been for me. When I first came to see you I could no longer run or jog due to generalized lack of cartilage in my right knee. An excellent orthopedic surgeon at Northwestern told me there was nothing traditional medicine could do to significantly improve my knee. And later, after taking the antibiotic Levaquin, I could no longer even take a running step.

I felt it would be a miracle if your Prolotherapy would allow me to run again. And after many treatments and exercise, that miracle has come to pass. I am once again jogging, playing hard tennis, and sprinting when want to. It is a remarkable change, and I once again feel physically complete and capable. Thanks sssooo much to you and your wonderful, friendly staff for bringing about this incredible cure. I highly recommend your services every chance I get."

*– Bill Adams**

"Several months ago my physical condition was so debilitated that I was issued a wheelchair. The arthritis in my left knee was so bad it caused excruciating pain. The usual treatments of steroid shots, non-inflammatory drugs, ice packs, etc. were of little use. In fact, I became progressively worse. Then I was advised the only help I could get was by having a knee-joint replacement. After months of tests, I was diagnosed with fibromyalgia, which is a painful condition affecting the muscles.

---

* Names have been changed to protect patients' privacy.

When the orthopedic doctor treating me received the report that I also suffered from fibromyalgia he compassionately informed me that he would not do a knee-joint replacement because I would not heal. He told me to consult my regular doctor for pain control. My physician informed me that he would prescribe medication to help me sleep as this is one of the serious affects of the condition.

Then, through an advertisement from a doctor believing in alternative, natural medicine, I first learned about Prolotherapy. Much to my surprise, when I called the 800 number in the advertisement, the gentleman referred me to Dr. Ross A. Hauser at Caring Medical and Rehabilitation Services in Oak Park, Illinois. My prayers were answered!

After just four treatments, my severely damaged knee-joint is healed. I am pain-free, except for some stiffness in the mornings which dissipates as I move about. Not only is Dr. Hauser a truly caring physician, but a godly man giving God the glory for the healing of his patients.

I wish to thank you, Dr. Hauser, and your compassionate staff for giving me, a 77 year old woman, a renewed life.

– Helen White*

"First of all, I'd like to thank you for returning the knee that God originally blessed me with fifty years ago (that's a heck of a warranty policy). After injuries in football, skydiving, and a number of other recreational sports, I limped onto the stage at The Natural USA Bodybuilding Championships in New York in 1993 and returned to the plane in a wheelchair! By God's grace I 'wheeled' away with the first place trophy in the Master's Division, but my knee was never the same.

I learned to live with pain, discomfort, and instability. Pickup games with my two boys in B-ball or football were no longer a consideration. Every step became a measured one and lateral movements were out of the question. Each morning I would descend our stairway one stair at a tie, have breakfast, read God's Word, and often pray for a new knee! My prayers were answered.

I received my fourth series of Prolotherapy shots a month ago and I walk pain free! I not only walk pain free, I run pain free. I cranked my treadmill up to seven miles an hour today and the only difficulty I had was sucking in enough oxygen! Since my initial visit I have sent twenty people to Caring Medical for Prolotherapy and success stories keep on coming.

Thank you for serving God with the gift that he has blessed you with, and for allowing so many of his children to be recipients of that gift as well.

– David Downs*

---

* Names have been changed to protect patients' privacy.

"When I first came to your office, I had terrible pain in my left knee. There was also a lot of swelling in the knee. I was sure that I needed knee surgery. A friend had recommended that I see you and I went in a very skeptical frame of mind. Having never heard of Prolotherapy I did not think that I could be cured by such a procedure. I decided to give you three or four months and if I was not better, then I would go ahead and get surgery. I had four treatments over a three month period. I have no pain in my knee, no swelling, and am back doing all the athletic sports that I enjoy. I cannot tell you how grateful I am for you and Prolotherapy. This is a procedure I would recommend to everyone and have already sent some of my friends to have you send their pain away. Thank you, thank you, thank you!"

– Mike Aaranov*

"On March 15, 2001 you treated my 15-year old daughter, Sharon,* with Prolotherapy. You gave her injections in her knees, where she has had chronic pain for nearly two years. Now, after one month and several days she is experiencing no pain in her knees and will be competing in a regional track meet this weekend, running the 800 meter run, the 1600 meter run and the 1600 meter relay. With the times she has logged in the past, she could be a major contender for the 800 meter run and hopefully will qualify to go our state track meet. Every day I ask her how her knees are and she says, 'Fine, I have no pain.' Being her mother, I ask, 'No pain—or are your knees just better?' And most emphatically she says, **'No pain.'** We are both thankful and grateful that we discovered you and Prolotherapy before we did something that could have caused permanent damage to her knees. We are telling everyone about our success with Prolotherapy and the supplements you prescribed on our visit there.

Thank you, thank you! I also want to tell you how much we appreciated the friendly, helpful people in your office."

– Alice Brownley*

"I came to see you about a very damaged knee. You administered Prolo to my knee and I feel great with my now good knees. I was able to win the World Jiu-Jitsu championships in 2001 and make it into the quarter finals in 2002. This is thought to be a young man's sport; I was competing against twenty year olds at the tender age of 46!

– Carl Kronen*

---

* Names have been changed to protect patients' privacy.

"I cannot tell you the joy I feel having no pain in my knees. I have had pain in my knees for many years. Doctors always prescribed anti-inflammatory drugs for over 10 years and were convinced I needed to have surgery to relieve the pain.

A very good friend told me about our procedure using Prolotherapy and I decided I had nothing to lose. I understood when you did the Prolotherapy that there was no guarantee I would be pain-free. I remember getting off the table after you administered the Prolotherapy injections and feeling no pain. I know from that day forward I have had no discomfort in my knees at all.

If you remember, my wife also received Prolotherapy from you on her shoulder. At that time she was suffering from a sprained rotator cuff and unable to raise her arm. After her Prolotherapy, she has had the same success as I.

I want to thank you again and if anyone ever questions your capabilities please have them call me!

*– Daniel Meijer**

I can't get those three years back in which I unnecessarily spent more time in doctors' offices and in physical therapy than I did in school, work, or life—but hopefully someone reading this can...

HOWARD WILLIAMS *

At the age of 26, Howard Williams had chronic back pain and was wearing permanent orthotic braces on both knees due to a several year run of what he feels to be bad luck. This young man was introduced to Prolotherapy, and his life has dramatically changed forever. The following is an excerpt from a letter Howard wrote to relay his gratitude:

"Today is October 28, 2003. I have had four treatments on my back with the fifth and final scheduled for next week, and it is cured. I have had thirteen treatments on my knees and I have been out of braces for four weeks. Both of my knee caps are back in place, the screw-home mechanism is fixed, neither leg is crooked, thus the muscle spasms have greatly dissipated. I still have a couple more treatments to do on my knees, but I am completely convinced I will get 100% recovery. I have literally felt my knees rotate back into place (no, not literally second-by-second, but month-to-month. I can tell the difference). As the legs have become more stable and in their proper alignment, the muscles have began to release and my physical therapist is able to work the painful scar tissue out, this time never to return. (When they break up the scar tissue, it feels like someone has poured rice crispies in my legs, and because the scar tissue causes the

---

* *Names have been changed to protect patients' privacy.*

muscles to lock up and prevents them from properly sliding fluidly across each other, it also feels like someone has poured glue, or marshmallows in my legs.)

This March will be the four-year anniversary of a knee sprain gone haywire because of bad orthopedic surgery. I know I am lucky to be walking today and am convinced I will be running by March. Even though I promised God that if he would just help me get my legs back I would never look back on this experience with anger, there is some anger. I am convinced that had the orthopedic community used Prolotherapy as a preemptive treatment before surgery, I would have walked into the office the week of my injury, received one or two treatments, and because nothing was torn but simply stretched over time, I would have been completely healed in a month. This would have been the same for my back and my left knee.

I can't get those three years back in which I unnecessarily spent more time in doctors' offices and in physical therapy than I did in school, work, or life—but hopefully someone reading this can. If you have been known to have patella problems, I hope you take this even more seriously. For as many doctors will tell you—people can walk and live an active life without other ligaments like the ACL or MCL—but when doctors go in and move your knee cap around, the implications can be disastrous.

I'll also be honest about the experience of actually getting the shots. It's no fun. Just think about it; you have a group of ligaments and connective tissue that is badly damaged and damaged tissue is sore and tender. On top of that, you have the tendons that are tender and inflamed because they are working overtime trying to stabilize the joints. Now, getting one flu shot in strong healthy shoulder tissue is no fun, but getting twenty-five in an inflamed knee is really not fun, but it's over in three minutes. If you're not willing to endure those three minutes of shots to end pain you've been living with for years, I call you foolish, but if you need help the doctor has means to ameliorate your experience.

As of the printing date of this book, Howard is done with his Prolotherapy sessions. He is running without braces—and more importantly—*without* pain. Yes, Howard is back to his game, and so can you with Prolotherapy! ■

Supplements for Your Prolotherapy

Many people are mistaken when they think that all supplements are the same. They are *not* the same—in fact I think you will be surprised at the difference in potency and quality on the market these days. Not all supplements are created equal.

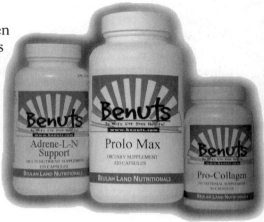

+ **More Potent**
+ **Better Quality**
+ **Accurate Labeling**

= **A better value for you!**

Value and Trust... this is what Beulah Land Nutritionals offers to each and every customer. Below is a Prolotherapy Enhancement Program recommended by Beulah Land Nutritionals. All of these products can be purchased at www.benuts.com.

BEULAH LAND NUTRITIONALS PROLOTHERAPY PROGRAM

PROLO MAX*
Prolo Max is used to help with soft tissue and connective tissue healing such as ligaments, tendons, and collagen. It may be used to help heal sports injuries, musculoskeletal pain and fibromyalgia.

BROMELAIN MAX*
Bromelain Max may be used to aid in soft tissue healing and acts as a natural pain reliever. Bromelain is made up of proteolytic enzymes that accelerate the inflammatory healing response, such as needed in the case of injury, degenerative joint disease, sports injury, chronic pain and can be used after Prolotherapy.

RAPID RESPONSE 1*
Rapid Response 1 is used to promote soft tissue healing and is helpful in conditions such as chronic pain, injuries, fibromyalgia, fatigue, joint stiffness and joint swelling.

SUPER OMEGA*

Super Omega is used to replace essential fatty acids, it is beneficial for arthritis, lubrication of joints, ligaments and tendons, and helps with the healing process of Prolotherapy.

COD LIVER OIL*

Cod Liver Oil is an excellent source of Omega 3 fatty acids and provides joint lubrication and assists in the healing process of Prolotherapy.

PRO CARTILAGE*

Pro Cartilage is used to rebuild cartilage and helps alleviate pain related to joint injury and arthritis.

PRO COLLAGEN*

Pro Collagen is used to re-build collagen and assists in the healing of soft tissue.

ENZYME MAX*

Enzyme Max is a high-potency enzyme preparation that speeds the the healing of soft tissue injuries. Athletes love this product. ■

Order your nutrition products online at:

www.benuts.com

Or, call us toll-free at:

877-RX-BEULAH

For a catalogue of the life-changing nutritional products available from Beulah Land Nutritionals, call in or e-mail us! (See next page for more information.)

---

* *The Food and Drug Administration have not evaluated the above statements. These products are not intended to diagnose, treat, cure or prevent any disease.*

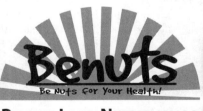
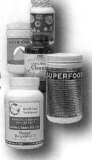

Other Books by Beulah Land Press

Beulah Land Press is pleased to offer these books on Prolotherapy written by Dr. Ross and Marion Hauser.

- *Prolo Your Pain Away!* Curing Chronic Pain with Prolotherapy
- *Prolo Your Sports Injuries Away!*
  Curing Sports Injuries and Enhancing Athletic Performance with Prolotherapy
- *Prolo Your Arthritis Pain Away!*
  Curing Disabling and Disfiguring Arthritis Pain with Prolotherapy
- *Prolo Your Back Pain Away!*
  Curing Chronic Back Pain with Prolotherapy
- *Prolo Your Headache and Neck Pain Away!*
  Curing Migraines and Neck Pain with Prolotherapy
- *Prolo Your Fibromyalgia Pain Away!*
  Curing Disabling Body Pain with Prolotherapy
- *Ligament and Tendon Relaxation Treated by Prolotherapy*
  By George S. Hackett, M.D., Gustav A. Hemwall, M.D., and Gerald A. Montgomery, M.D.

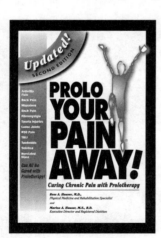

ABOUT THESE BOOKS:
PROLO YOUR PAIN AWAY!

Read the book that has changed chronic pain management forever. "This is the best book ever written about Prolotherapy," says Robert C. Atkins, M.D., best-selling author of *New Diet Revolution* and medical director of the Atkins Center for Complementary Medicine in New York City, New York. *Prolo Your Pain Away!* details in common lay language the conditions that can be cured with Prolotherapy, including arthritis, back pain, migraines, neck pain, fibromyalgia, spastic torticollis, osteoporosis, fracture pain, cancer pain, whiplash, sports injuries, loose joints, TMJ, tendonitis, sciatica, herniated discs, and more! Find out why C. Everett Koop, M.D., former Surgeon General of the United States, and a former chronic pain sufferer who was cured by Prolotherapy, says *"Prolo Your Pain Away!* is a must-read for anyone experiencing chronic musculoskeletal pain."

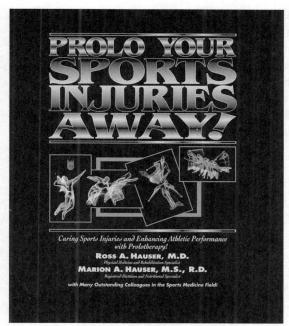

Curing Sports Injuries and Enhancing Athletic Performance with Prolotherapy!
ROSS A. HAUSER, M.D.
Physical Medicine and Rehabilitation Specialist
MARION A. HAUSER, M.S., R.D.
Registered Dietitian and Nutritional Specialist
with Many Outstanding Colleagues in the Sports Medicine Field!

PROLO YOUR SPORTS INJURIES AWAY!

Just as the original book *Prolo Your Pain Away!* affected the pain management field, *Prolo Your Sports Injuries Away!* has rattled the sports world. Learn the 20 myths of sports medicine, including the myths of anti-inflammatory medications; why cortisone shots actually weaken tissue; how ice, rest, and immobilization may actually hurt the athlete; why the common practice of taping and bracing does not stabilize injured areas; and why the arthroscope is one of the athlete's worst nightmares!

Did you ever wonder why most career runners and athletes end up with arthritis? This book will explain why this happens and how you can prevent it from happening to you! Prolotherapy is an athlete's best friend because it addresses the root cause of most sports injuries: ligament and tendon weakness. By stimulating the body to repair the painful area, Prolotherapy can make an injured area stronger than its original, uninjured counterpart! Athletes around the country are hailing Prolotherapy as the treatment that not only added more years to their careers, but also gave them that additional edge by enhancing their athletic performance. You will learn why Prolotherapy has become the sports medicine treatment of the future and why athletes around the country are curing their sports injuries and enhancing their athletic performance with Prolotherapy.

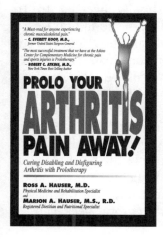

"A Must-read for anyone experiencing chronic musculoskeletal pain."
— C. EVERETT KOOP, M.D.,
former United States Surgeon General

"The most successful treatment that we have at the Atkins Center for Complementary Medicine for chronic pain and sports injuries is Prolotherapy."
— ROBERT C. ATKINS, M.D.,
New York Times Best-Selling Author

PROLO YOUR ARTHRITIS PAIN AWAY!
Curing Disabling and Disfiguring Arthritis with Prolotherapy

ROSS A. HAUSER, M.D.
Physical Medicine and Rehabilitation Specialist
and
MARION A. HAUSER, M.S., R.D.
Registered Dietitian and Nutritional Specialist

PROLO YOUR ARTHRITIS PAIN AWAY!

Studies estimate that 40 million people in the United States suffer from some form of arthritis. By the year 2020 that number will be nearly 60 million. The traditional treatments for arthritis involve anti-inflammatory medication, cortisone shots, and joint replacement surgery. People are often left with the diagnosis of: "There is nothing else we can do for you." Nothing could be further from the truth. What most people do not realize is that arthritis forms because of an underlying ligament and joint weakness problem. The body responds to this weakness by overgrowing bony formations in the unstable areas, hoping to provide some stabilization to the weak joint. Unfortunately, this is not only painful, but often disfiguring.

Prolotherapy is the best technique available to stimulate the body to strengthen the joint and surrounding ligaments. By doing this, the arthritis process stops and the pain can be eliminated. This book details why arthritis sufferers around the country are throwing away the anti-inflammatory medications and returning to the activities that they used to enjoy. Prolotherapy has given life back to many arthritis sufferers. Gone are the days of waking up feeling stiff and sore.

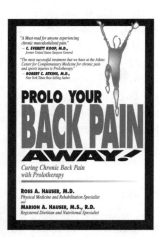

PROLO YOUR BACK PAIN AWAY!

Stan Mikita, former Chicago Blackhawks hockey star and hall-of-famer, was about to cut a magnificent career short because of a back injury. Six weeks prior to the 1971-1972 season opening, Mr. Mikita could not even get out of bed because of severe sciatica and back pain. He found Prolotherapy as a treatment option that got him back on his skates again. Learn why Stan enthusiastically says, "Prolotherapy definitely extended my NHL career eight years and gave me complete relief of my back pain!" Learn why MRI scans may erroneously diagnose "disc problems," forcing people into unnecessary surgeries. Prolotherapy can help the painful conditions such as degenerated disc disease, sciatica, arthritis, spinal stenosis, and even herniated discs. This is why people with chronic back pain are saying "no" to surgery and "yes" to Prolotherapy!

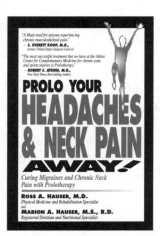

PROLO YOUR HEADACHE AND NECK PAIN AWAY!

Years ago, it was going to be another ruined evening for the Hausers. Marion had another migraine headache. She finally decided to try Prolotherapy to put an end to the suffering. Boy, is she glad that she did! You will also be glad if you suffer from migraines, tension, or cluster headaches. Marion went from being a skeptic to someone who now writes books on the topic! Prolotherapy stimulates the body to repair painful areas. Don't most headaches start out with neck or shoulder pain? Learn about a lesser-known syndrome called Barré-Lieou Syndrome, which is one of the most common causes of headaches. Some of the associated symptoms include ringing in the ears, sinus pressure, dizziness, and neck pain. Ligament injury in the neck is usually the cause of head-forward posture, which leads to chronic neck pain and headaches. Prolotherapy causes the vertebrae in the neck to stay in alignment. Good alignment means good posture. Good posture means fewer headaches. No more headaches mean good-bye to pain pills. Learn why many former headache sufferers found hope with Prolotherapy.

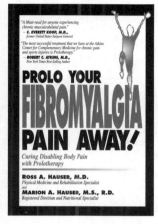

PROLO YOUR FIBROMYALGIA PAIN AWAY!

An epidemic number of people in the United States wake up in the morning feeling tired, sore, and achy. Upon physical examination, tender points are found all over the body. Women may be given the concurrent diagnoses of migraine headaches and endometriosis. They are told to exercise and take antidepressant medication. Nothing can be done to cure the problem... until now. Learn why over 90 percent of fibromyalgia sufferers respond well to Prolotherapy. People with Fibromyalgia often suffer from fungal infections, which have a tremendously detrimental effect on soft tissue formation, including the ligaments and tendons. Treatment of this infection, in conjunction with Prolotherapy, has given hope to many suffering from the often-debilitating symptoms of fibromyalgia.

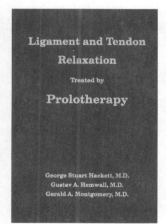

LIGAMENT AND TENDON RELAXATION TREATED BY PROLOTHERAPY

After performing Prolotherapy for over 40 years, the world's most experienced Prolotherapist, Gustav A. Hemwall, M.D., died at the age of 90. His legacy and experience are preserved in this fifth edition of the book written by the originator himself, George S. Hackett, M.D. Dr. Hackett wrote many of the words in this book. This book was written to demonstrate the technique of Prolotherapy to physicians. Many case studies are also presented. Much of what is known about Prolotherapy comes from the authors of this book

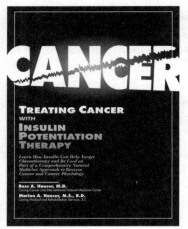

TREATING CANCER WITH INSULIN POTENTIATION THERAPY

Learn How Insulin Can Be Used As Part of a Comprehensive Program To Reverse Cancer and Cancer Physiology

Insulin Potentiation Therapy (IPT) is an effective and powerful treatment for cancer. IPT uses Insulin to increase the cancer-killing effects of chemotherapy. Because of this "potentiating" effect, lower doses of chemotherapy are used, making it a much safer option than traditional methods in the treatment of cancer.

IPT was first used by its originator, Dr. Donato Perez Garcia, of Mexico, in 1934. Despite numerous successes in the cure of many infectious diseases and cancers, the treatment was largely ignored by the medical profession. Dr. Perez Garcia was able to pass his knowledge down to his son Dr. Donato Garcia y Bellon, who subsequently taught it to his son, Dr. Donato Perez Garcia, who now practices in Tijuana, Mexico.

IPT as part of a comprehensive natural medicine program. Treating Cancer with Insulin Potentiation Therapy is not just about using IPT to treat cancer. IPT, diet, and natural medicine help reverse "cancer physiology" which allowed the cancer to start and thrive in the first place. This approach to cancer gets at the probable causes of the cancer, making it a very science-based, integrative, safe, and often curative, treatment option for the cancer patient. ■

PURCHASING INFORMATION
Beulah Land Press • 715 Lake Street
Oak Park, Illinois 60301
1-800-RX-PROLO (1-800-797-7656)
www.benuts.com • www.beulahlandpress.com

For Further Information
www.caringmedical.com • www.proloinfo.com

INDEX

181